THE
ALZHEIMER'S
HANDBOOK

THE
ALZHEIMER'S
HANDBOOK

*A guide to the diagnosis and
management of the causes of
confusion and dementia*

Professor Gerry Bennett
and Dr Mark Jones

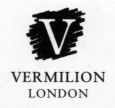

VERMILION
LONDON

1 3 5 7 9 10 8 6 4 2

Text © Gerry Bennett and Mark Jones 2001

Gerry Bennett and Mark Jones have asserted their moral rights
to be identified as the authors of this work under the
Copyright, Designs and Patent Act 1988.

First published in the United Kingdom in 1989
by Macdonald Optima
This revised edition published in 2001 by Vermilion,
an imprint of Ebury Press, Random House,
20 Vauxhall Bridge Road, London SW1V 2SA

Random House Australia (Pty) Limited
20 Alfred Street, Milsons Point, Sydney,
New South Wales 2061, Australia

Random House New Zealand Limited
18 Poland Road, Glenfield, Auckland 10, New Zealand

Random House South Africa (Pty) Limited
Endulini, 5A Jubilee Road, Parktown 2193, South Africa

The Random House Group Limited Reg. No. 954009

Papers used by Vermilion are natural, recyclable products
made from wood grown in sustainable forests.

Printed and bound in Great Britain
by Mackays of Chatham Ltd, Chatham, Kent

A CIP catalogue record for this book is available from the
British Library.

ISBN 0 09 185738 4

Contents

Introduction

By the year 2020 it is estimated that one quarter of the population will be of retirement age. Increased life expectancy is, however, a double-edged sword. Society is youth and work orientated, and the mental and physical frailty that may accompany ageing is increasingly having to be managed by medicine and the social services. On the other hand, while retirement for many means loss of role and status, because of the social and medical advances of the last hundred years we are fitter and healthier than we have ever been. The ageing brain is now becoming a social and medical challenge. Patients and their relatives are often surprised by the catastrophic impact that abnormal mental processes can produce in someone they have known and loved for a lifetime and who was physically and mentally well in their life to date. The patient is perplexed and frightened, the family is fearful and does not know how to go about asking for help. Being old can then be a terrible experience. The world in which today's elderly grew up and worked now moves at a very different pace. Isolation is a profound problem, and a contented old age is very much dependent upon enough social contacts, good housing and adequate finances. Until recently people gave little thought to planning their retirement, but the state pension is inadequate for quality living, although it is what many of this country's older people depend upon. The Government, conscious of the growing challenge of an ageing population is anxious that more people have some form of top up pension.

The health and social requirements of elderly people can be complex and, hitherto, have been an unfashionable branch of medicine. This, fortunately, has changed over the last 20 years, particularly with specific training at senior levels in the medical (including psychiatric) and social work professions. There are many committed individuals who have chosen to advance the notion that being old need not have dire consequences. 'Treatments' have become 'packages of care' reviewing all aspects of a patient's life. Wear and tear is inevitable, but the expectations that *all* elderly persons will become confused, immobile and incontinent, or simply unable to cope ('acopia' as it is known in accident and emergency departments) is simply false. The body has enormous capacity to cope and adapt to adverse circumstances. The psychology of ageing is now a focus of much research and practical help is available. Attitudes and services are evolving but pejorative terms such as 'geriatric' or, even worse, 'crumble' are still commonplace. National Health Service budgets are inevitably soaring, and it is those with a voice and a comparatively longer productive life who get the best deals. Where you live has, to some extent, determined the quality of healthcare you receive, and today post code rationing of newer and costly treatments is commonplace. Yet patients are getting to know what they are entitled to, partly fuelled by a better-informed media-led society. There remain, however, many that suffer indignities of social and medical neglect and have not the voice or know-how to remedy their situation.

This book is aimed at patients, carers and healthcare workers who do not want a textbook but a practical guide to acute and chronic confusional states. We hope it will give them the information they need to understand what they are facing and how to access the relevant services. The book is divided broadly into sections on the types of condition that cause confusion, other conditions that can cause confusional states, how to access services and what you can expect in terms of management and possible treatments, including the most recent information on drugs known collectively as the acetylcholinesterase inhibitors. There is also a section on the legal aspects of how to manage the affairs of a person who has become confused. Institutional care is sometimes inevitable despite the best care and efforts of everyone involved, so specific information on this has been included. There are many sufferers of Alzheimer's disease and related conditions whose lives have been made not just bearable but who have been allowed a quality of life that previously was thought unworthy of investment. In its most malignant form Alzheimer's is a devastating and tragic condition, but that is not to say that there is not a system out there which can support the patient and the family through this difficult journey. We believe that our working lives have been well spent in helping to develop these services and caring for an unfairly neglected section of society.

1

The Old Age Revolution

If statistics alone were the proof of success then old age would be a sure-fire winner. A hundred years ago about four per cent of the population were aged 65 or over. This figure is now about 18 per cent or roughly eight million elderly people. How has this explosion in numbers come about? It is the result of a set of complex and intermingled factors. Since the beginning of the last century especially, our basic living conditions have greatly improved and the majority of us now take for granted piped hot and cold water, flushing toilets, homes with lighting and heating, and fairly unlimited basic food provision. This said, too many older people still live in poverty, dependent on inadequate state resources, but for the majority of us the improvement in our social and physical environment has meant that our general health has also improved. We no longer suffer the ravages of epidemics such as cholera and bubonic plague, which were commonplace in grossly insanitary and over-crowded conditions only a few generations ago.

Medical advances

Advances in medicine have played a less dramatic role in this increased surge in numbers of older people. Sophisticated health services ensure that people do not die of common conditions such as appendicitis or complicated bone fractures, as used to be the case. We now take for granted antibiotics, anaesthesia for operations, and even spare-part surgery. Although trends are for families to have fewer children, virtually all of them will live to be old and many to be very old indeed. Most babies now born in the United Kingdom, Europe and the developed world can confidently expect to live to around 80 years of age. Obviously the total number of older people in a population will depend on the birth rate many years previously and any special factors, such as wars, that may have intervened.

The demographics of age

The end of the 20th century saw interesting changes in the age distribution of the population. The total number of older people peaked, and a cohort (i.e. well-defined group) of old old (85+) also rose substantially. These people were born before the First World War and though suffering the ravages of war and influenza epidemic also reaped the benefits of the social and medical changes that increased their life expectancy. However, the First World War will also be remembered for removing a generation of young men, leaving a large number of women to remain unmarried or widowed, hence entering their old age much more isolated. A small but significant number of these women (and a few men) are our current centenarians. Life expectancy continued to rise throughout the last century and into this one, posing a profound challenge for our society.

The next challenge is close at hand. Following the Second World War there was a surge in births, the so-called 'baby boomers'. This bulge of humanity will reach the age of 65 from 2010 onwards, peaking over the next decade. The interesting phenomenon here will be not only the numbers involved but also their attitudes to health, ageing, services and politics. This group have had it all – peace, prosperity, rising living standards, decreasing poverty and a consumer led service economy. The majority will be more affluent, articulate and politically powerful than the widows and spinsters of the end of the century before (who were present at the birth of health and social services).

The new challenge

The issue we face therefore is the growing number of older people who will make increasingly greater demands on our health and social services. People are much more health conscious, they will want to see their general practitioner and other members of the primary care team more frequently. When admission is necessary they will probably be spending longer in hospital and need more complex multidisciplinary assessment. In the community, where the largest proportion of older people are always to be found, the most frail will need increased amounts of support from specialist housing, social services and the private and voluntary sector. The needs of their carers must also be met. The oldest old (85+) will have the highest proportion of physical and mental frailty and, although a relatively small proportion of the total number of old people, this group will require a larger share of available resources if their needs are to be adequately covered.

The health and care needs of older people increasingly occupy the minds of politicians. In the UK we have had notice of these trends for many decades, and as our total population is relatively stable and birth and death rates are monitored, our governments have had long periods for planning. Limitless demand and cost, however, have led to innovative ways of tackling health and social issues such as care in the community and primary care led services, including the concept of intermediate care and telephone helplines to screen enquiries (which we will deal with later).

Consider for a moment what is happening in developing countries, many of which have had high birth rates – sometimes tacitly encouraged by governments to meet labour demands – disease and the social ills of poverty. Developed world technology, and to some extent values, rapidly changed people's aspirations. Birth rates fell dramatically, and increased prosperity also improved living standards. Within the span of one generation these countries have been faced with a huge number of young people growing old and living into advanced old age. Government health and social planning in these circumstances takes on a truly different meaning. In the developing world the pace of change means that they are looking at the mistakes the developed world made and striving not to replicate them. The concept of institutions for older people is alien to the cultures of many of these countries and large-scale provision is financially impossible. Many countries are spending what limited resources they have on prevention of the conditions that afflict elders and on keeping elderly people in the community, using modern teaching methods and health care technology to promote primary care services and community health policies.

If meeting the needs of a large number of very old people is a challenge, then meeting the needs of that group suffering from chronic confusion is difficult indeed. Taken at face value the numbers seem enormous and overwhelming; even a multidisciplinary advisory group not used to overstatement once called the impending challenge 'the rising tide'. The facts as they are known indicate that when the numbers of the very old are at their peak there will be over one million old people in the United Kingdom with some form of dementia. This represents about one in ten of the total number of over 65s and one in five of the very old i.e. 85+.

The numbers involved will cause formidable difficulties unless truly seamless and accessible services are further developed and organised now. Society as a whole, and the health and social services in particular, are not coping with the current number of old people, especially those with dementia. Until the mid-1980s only six per cent of elderly people in the UK lived in any form of institution such as old people's homes or hospital long-term care wards. This was one of the lowest figures for institutional care in the developed world. The need for care, in some form, was obviously not being met, however, and when the then Conservative government decided to pay for residential or nursing home care without compulsory assessment the flood gates opened. The cost was soon counted in billions of pounds. The situation could not continue, and (without electoral discussion) the cost of placement was transferred to the older person as a call on any assets they might have. There are now nearly 200,000 nursing home beds alone, an increase of 300 per cent, with a dramatic decrease in hospital provision. About eight per cent of people over 65 are now in institutional care. The lifetime 'risk' of entry into a care home is about 20 per cent for a man aged 65 and 36 per cent for a women. The debate over who should pay is now as fierce as ever, with changes just announced by the Labour government.

The majority of older people live in their own homes, many helped by their families, and at least a quarter live alone. The UK was once looked upon as a world leader in its range of provision for elderly people. That is sadly no longer the case. The provision is breaking down and basic services that ensure a minimum quality of life and keep an individual at home with some form of independence and dignity are not being delivered. There are insufficient services for the elderly mentally frail and their carers, and few have access to day and night sitting services or respite care. Our institutions, when they have to be used, remain under-staffed and under-resourced. Carers, be they family or otherwise, keep our system from collapsing about our ears; they are the group that continue to face daily burdens. We fail them as we fail the older person – at our peril.

The fact that life expectancy continues to rise is surely the success story of the last and hopefully this millennium. It is now comparatively common for someone to live to be 100 though it is still far from the norm. Some scientists believe that we are approaching the limit of life expectancy for most of us and that the few that surpass it by many years are in fact 'biologically elite'. They feel that we are genetically pro-grammed to self-destruct at a certain age and that social and health trends cannot continue to extend the human lifespan. Many others feel that we are at the beginning of one of the greatest periods in our evolution and that we are only just starting on the journey of increasing our lifespan. Research work on flies, mice and rats suggests that we can prolong their life expectancy considerably. The study of ageing – gerontology – is now a rapidly expanding field of scientific research. It has finally shed its image of quacks searching for the elixir of youth and is beginning to show that the ageing process is far more complicated than was previously thought. The new knowledge of the genetic structure of our genes down to the enzymes that appear to control ageing within cells means that immortality is no longer science fiction, though aiming for routine ages of 150 is a more realistically next achievable step.

Whatever the outcome of this research, older people are destined to be the social and health focus for the early part of this new millennium. We must strive to ensure that quality of life rather than quantity remains the overriding principle – 'add life to years'.

2

Acute Confusion

Acute confusion in older people is a remarkably common condition. 'Acute' can mean anything from a confused state lasting only a few minutes to a state lasting a few months, although the majority of episodes of confusion are short-lived. The point that must be stressed, however, is that confusion does not mean dementia and that acute confusion occurring in an older person is simply a way of presenting an underlying illness process. The vast majority of apparently acute confusional states are fully reversible.

What do we mean by acute confusion? One of the best descriptive words for it is 'delirium'. One can then picture the sufferer being disorientated in time and place; they are not sure where they are or what time of day it is. Their 'feeling state' is up and down, one minute they are calm and happy to co-operate, and the next they are agitated and wanting to do inappropriate things. The person's memory is usually poor, and they can be quite drowsy at times. One of the most distressing features is the tendency to hallucinate and suffer delusions. In this situation what a psychiatrist calls 'affect' means that the patient is often perplexed, anxious and fearful. The mood is often labile, i.e. the patient can rapidly go from tears to laughter.

Hallucinations occur more commonly if the person has poor eyesight and hearing but also tend to happen when the light is poor (during the twilight times of dawn and evening). The condition of confusion occurring at twilight has been termed 'sun downing' syndrome. It is also common for objects to get mistaken for something else – the pattern on the carpet becomes a mass of crawling insects. Delusions are false ideas that the deluded person will not accept as wrong and which are not amenable to reason; you can talk and explain until you are blue in the face but the person will still insist that they are right. Delusions can take many forms and in acute confusion they are usually short-lived, with periods of normal thinking. They may be slightly comical to family or onlookers – for example, the sufferer may insist that a number 48 bus is due in their bedroom any minute to take them to the shops, hence they cannot leave – but they are invariably distressing, especially if the person insists, for example, that their food is poisoned or that one of their carers is going to harm them. These are known as paranoid delusions, paranoia being a mental state where you wrongly think that you yourself or others are going to be harmed.

People with acute confusional states are not usually aggressive but often agitated. Occasionally violence in the form of hitting out occurs, usually as the result of the con-fused person being restrained from doing something which is potentially harmful for them. If the person is agitated, their speech is often affected and sentences don't get finished as they rush onto something else; on the other hand, drows-iness can make their speech a little slurred. Conditions that cause confusional states to come on very suddenly (such as infections) often cause the person to look and feel unwell. They may be flushed and warm to the touch, even sweating. They may complain of vague aches and pains as well as having no appetite. Nausea and vomiting can occur and the confusion may be accompanied by weakness and lethargy. Sometimes no other symptoms occur and yet an underlying illness is still present.

You will realise from what has been described above that these conditions can be very frightening for carers. Suddenly they may be dealing with a relative who not only appears unwell but is also difficult to handle, control and comfort. The confusion may be accompanied by the other symptoms (for example, weakness or incontinence). The carer may be accused of nasty deeds, or have a difficult job stopping their relative trying to leave the house or doing other inappropriate acts. Sometimes it is nothing as florid as the above descriptions, just a feeling on the part of the carers that all is not right and that the older person, in some hard to define way, is not their usual self. This usually stems from some odd behaviour or speech, which indicates that the person is confused.

Acute confusional states can also occur in a person with chronic dementia. The causes are usually the same, and the stable baseline state is interrupted by a sudden worsening of faculties which, when the condition is treated, remits allowing the person to return to their stable state again.

Causes of acute confusion

The following list indicates some of the more common causes of acute confusion in older people. The main ones are discussed in more detail explaining the condition, how they might be diagnosed (recognised) by carer and doctor and finally how they are treated:

• urinary tract infection
• chest infection
• drugs
• stroke
• heart attack
• severe diarrhoea and vomiting (gastro-enteritis)
• chronic skin wounds (leg ulcers and pressure sores)
• sugar diabetes

In the very frail the following can also precipitate an acute confusional state:

- moving house/admission to sheltered housing or residential or nursing home
- admission to/discharge from hospital
- accidental fall
- bereavement
- failing eyesight and hearing

Urinary tract infection

This is a very common condition especially in older women. When it occurs in men it is often associated with an enlarged prostate gland (see diagram opposite) which makes it harder to pass urine. There are many reasons why urinary tract infections are more common in older women. The short passage from the bladder to the outside (see diagram opposite) means that infection can easily and quickly enter the bladder, particularly if the area between the bottom and the front passage is not kept especially clean. This can happen if a woman wipes her bottom forwards, soiling the front passage and introducing infection. Also, as a woman gets older she produces less of the hormones (oestrogen) which usually keep the vagina lubricated. Thus the front passage can get dry and sore, and infection can occur more easily. Infections of all kinds occur more often if the person has sugar diabetes. Drinking insufficient liquid (dehydration) leads to a poor urine flow, which may also cause an increased tendency to infection.

Apart from confusion there are other ways in which a urinary tract infection can show itself. The urine may smell strongly and be quite offensive. It may also hurt to pass it, causing a burning sensation. Urinary tract infections commonly cause incontinence, in which case the infected urine can be detected by carers. Occasionally, in a woman, the infection may be so severe as to make it impossible to pass urine; the bladder becomes painfully full and only small amounts of urine leak out. This is called retention and is

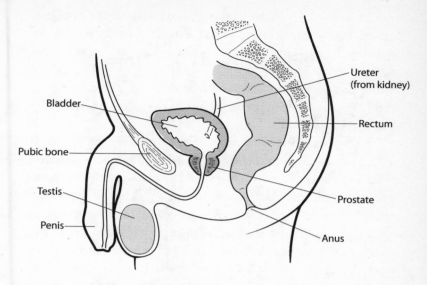

The male urinary and genital systems

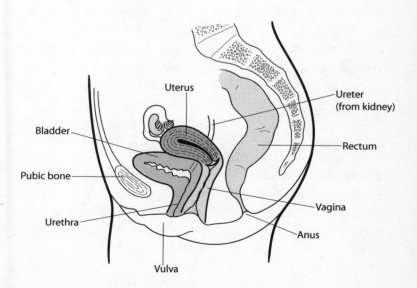

The female urinary and genital systems

more usually seen in men when the prostate gland gets to a size that blocks the flow of urine. Rarely, an infection causes a lot of blood in the urine, which is always a sign that medical help should be sought.

Prevention is obviously the best cure, and good hygiene can help a lot. Many people believe that a good supply of fluids, especially fruit juice (some specialists recommend cranberry juice) helps to prevent urinary tract infections. If there is a severe hormone lack (this usually needs a gentle examination of the front passage by a doctor or specialist nurse to confirm it) then some locally applied hormone cream is very effective. In most cases of established infection a short course of antibiotics will cure it. The doctor or nurse may dip the urine for blood and protein (as well as substances called nitrites) which are present in infected urine, and many will collect a recently passed sample to send to the laboratory to grow the bugs responsible and ensure that the antibiotics are effective. However, if the affected person is incontinent and there are troubling features present it is best to start treatment immediately. If the older person is very unwell (toxic or unable to pass water) then admission to hospital may be necessary.

For further information see Appendix 1, page 171.

Chest infection

Chest infections occur more commonly in winter, especially if the lungs are already diseased. Smoking is the main cause of lung damage and causes the conditions of chronic bronchitis and emphysema (breathing difficulties with shortness of breath, cough and phlegm) as well as lung cancer. People with these conditions get much worse symptoms when a chest infection occurs, so smoking should be stopped if at all possible at any age, no matter how few cigarettes are being smoked. An older person's lungs may have been affected by their occupation – for example, coal mining – or exposure to asbestos or other forms of dust. Lungs may be weakened by other chronic diseases such as asthma, operations, complications of old tuberculosis (TB) infection, or – now very rarely (so few of these men are still alive) – gassing in the First World War. Even healthy lungs can become infected. Influenza epidemics are particularly dangerous for older people, especially those with a pre-existing lung or general health problem.

Chest infections can be difficult to diagnose early. Diagnosis becomes easier if any mental confusion is accompanied by a cough, especially a fruity one, and the person can cough up phlegm. Phlegm (secretions usually produced in the lungs and swallowed without noticing) can be coughed up in normal circumstances, when it is clear or white. In a chest infection it becomes green or yellow and may, rarely, contain some blood. The infection may be accompanied by some chest pains; when these occur on deep breathing it is suggestive of pleurisy (inflammation of the lining of the lungs and chest wall). The earliest sign that a chest infection is present is often breathlessness. This may not be complained of but the carer may notice that at the beginning of the illness the person is breathing quite fast and shallowly while sitting at rest.

Chest infections are caused either by bacteria or by viruses. In bacterial infections antibiotics are needed to kill the bugs. Smoking should be stopped. Sometimes the infection is accompanied by wheezing, in which case other drugs (often in inhaler or vapour form) are given. Coughing helps bring up the secretions (which can be copious) and is therefore a good thing. However, it can sometimes be exhausting and painful and needs to be lessened (usually with a codeine-based linctus). People with already damaged lungs may need the help of home oxygen during a new infection, but this should always be supervised at the start by a doctor, as some patients cannot tolerate oxygen. Some areas of the country have physiotherapists who visit people at home and help them clear the congested lungs by tapping firmly on the chest whilst putting the patient in different positions.

Influenza is caused by a virus. Unlike bacteria, viruses are not killed by antibiotics, so antibiotics should not be routinely prescribed unless complications occur (such as bacterial pneumonia). Instead, treatment is supportive and along the lines stated above. It is possible, however, to offer some protection against influenza by vaccination. The injections are available to older people from their GP from September onwards, and they are especially recommended for the very frail and those with existing lung damage. New anti-viral influenza tablets are also now available from GPs. They need to be started as soon as possible after the symptoms start. As with urinary tract infections, if the condition is serious then admission to hospital becomes necessary.

Drugs

Older people as a group are enormous consumers of prescription and over-the-counter drugs, as well as remedies from health food shops. However, it is only recently that any new drugs have been tried out in their research stage in clinical trials on older subjects. Such clinical trials are important because it is now well known that older people respond to drugs differently than younger adults. Drugs are broken down in the body or changed into different forms and even stored in the fat, but ultimately have to be got rid of. This can be via the liver, mixed with bile, or in the urine, or even by sweat and breath. The way in which drugs are dealt with by the body is extremely relevant because as we age our kidneys especially become less efficient. There is thus a risk of drug build-up in the blood stream. If this happens, instead of doing good the drug begins to cause harm, and one way this can show itself is in the person becoming confused.

The dose of the drug is therefore very important and for most older people it should be the smallest dose possible to give the desired effect. A good example of this problem is the heart drug Digoxin. This drug is used where the heart-beat is irregular (usually atrial fibrillation) and is going too fast. The drug slows the heart down. The usual dose for this drug in young adults is 0.25mg (250mcg). This has been found over the years of use to be far too strong for most older people, as it is cleared by the kidneys and tends to build up in the blood stream, causing nausea and vomiting and heart problems of its own. A smaller dose of 0.125 mg (125mcg) was made available but even this proved to be too high a dose for most older people; thus a 0.0625mg (62.5mcg) dose was established, called the P/G dose (paed-iatric/geriatric). Digoxin is also a good example of another drug phenomenon, the therapeutic window. This is the level of drug in the blood to give the best effect. For Digoxin it is a measurement of between 1 and 2 (mg/ml) i.e. below 1 and the drug is not working; between 1 and 2 it is effective; over 2 it causes side effects. So its therapeutic window is very narrow, which makes the use of the drug more complicated.

The time a drug takes to be eliminated from the body is called its half-life; drugs that take a long time to be got rid of are said to have a long half-life. Because an older person's kidneys are less efficient it can be seen that those drugs with long half-lives are potentially the most dangerous. An example of this problem is the group of drugs known as tranquillisers and night sedatives. One of largest groups is the benzodiazepines (i.e. Diazepam, Temazepam, etc.). They are used to induce sleep or make a person less anxious. They have many unwanted side effects, including dependence, but one of the group – nitrazepam – has special problems for older people. It has a very long half-life in some older people so that the acting level of the drug gradually builds up and causes drowsiness by day, unsteadiness and a tendency to fall, as well as confusion. All sedatives and tranquillisers have the risk of inducing falls and confusion in older people and must therefore be used with caution. Nitrazepam should not be used at all.

If a single drug can cause symptoms of confusion, a cocktail of five or six different drugs almost guarantees it. It is a feature of illness in old age that there are multiple problems, and some or all may require drug therapy. It is also true, however, that (like younger patients) elderly people do not need to stay on a specific drug for very long. Only rarely do drugs have to be given continuously, and even then the dosage can usually be reduced over time. If an older person is given five or six drugs in hospital then, if at all possible, they should be down to at least three by the date of discharge. The GP can usually safely reduce them still further, only re-introducing a drug if the person's condition relapses. Multiple drug therapy leads to poor compliance (that is, drugs just don't get taken), drug interactions causing unwanted side effects and, if not monitored, a continuation of some drugs when they are not needed. Repeat prescriptions in older people should be regularly reviewed by GPs before automatic reissuing.

Some drugs are well known for their ability to cause confusion in older people. If these need to be prescribed, the patient and carers need appropriate information so that they can be on their guard and contact their doctor early if confusion does occur. All of the drugs used to treat Parkinson's disease can cause confusion, especially a group of drugs called the anticholinesterases, for example benzhexol and drugs containing L-dopa. The side effects of these drugs are usually reversible by lowering the dose or stopping the drug under a doctor's guidance. Steroids are very powerful drugs used for treating many conditions including asthma, inflammatory conditions and cancer. These drugs must never be stopped suddenly and so, if confusion occurs, a doctor must advise on the best course of action. Water tablets (diuretics) are used in the treatment of heart failure when there is an excess of fluid in the body due to the heart's pump action being impaired. The drugs can be gentle or very powerful but all have the potential to deplete the body of salts (sodium and potassium), and if they are taken for too long or in too high a dose they can cause dehydration. Both these side effects can cause symptoms of confusion in the older person. Rarely they are given (or taken) for the wrong reasons, such as to decrease the size of swollen legs or ankles or to cause weight loss. They should not be used for either (swollen legs in elderly people is usually due to immobility or not going to bed, and the legs should be raised up as much as is tolerated).

Drugs should always be suspected when a confusional state occurs. It is likely that almost any drug can cause confusion so they must all be regarded with suspicion. When a drug is prescribed, both doctor and patient should be clear as to why the drug is being given, how long the course of treatment will be and what are the possible side effects. It is an excellent plan for GPs to issue older people prescription cards or sheets listing current medication, dose and length of course. Hospital admission often results in new medication. Ideally the same drug card should be used so that both patient and GP know what new medication has been given from the day of discharge.

Stroke

To most people a stroke means sudden weakness down one side of the body due to a clot of blood in the brain. The weakness is often associated with many other problems including speech disturbance, difficulty swallowing, incontinence and the dangers of sudden immobility. In fact there are many types and causes of stroke. Full-blown stroke, where the weakness is very obvious, can be due to a large clot of blood (an embolus), but it is most commonly caused by a gradual furring up of an important blood vessel; in the end the remaining narrow passage blocks and no more blood can reach that bit of the brain (this is called an infarct – the brain is starved of oxygen as the heart is in a heart attack). Occasionally a stroke is due to a blood vessel rupturing (like the blow out of a car tyre) and blood pouring into the brain and causing damage (a haemorrhage). In this type of stroke there can be a history of high blood pressure. All of the above types of stroke can happen quite quickly, though usually a haemorrhagic stroke is the most rapid and an infarct can evolve over some hours. All the types of stroke can be fatal. The many who survive often take weeks or months to recover the use of their limbs and/or speech.

It is now recognised that not all strokes are as major as the ones described above. In older people especially, small strokes can occur without any major weakness of the arms or legs being noticed. It is thought that the furred-up vessels in the body cause very small clots of blood to form (because the blood flow becomes disturbed over the bumps). These small clots get carried to the brain. If they are big enough they can cause slight weakness of an arm or leg (or both) or a slight speech disturbance such as slurred speech with a drooping mouth, but this usually goes within 24 hours. Sometimes these small areas of damage cause no weakness at all but can make the person confused. This too often passes quite quickly, but the whole process recurs, sometimes accompanied by limb weakness, blackouts or falls. This condition can be difficult to diagnose unless some obvious signs of a stroke occur.

These repeated mini-stokes are called transient ischaemic attacks (TIAs) – the term means short-lived blockage in the blood supply – and are important for many reasons. They sometimes occur before a major stroke and can act as a warning so that treatable causes of major strokes can be looked for. A fairly common condition is the furring up of the main arteries in the neck (the carotid arteries) which supply the brain. These can need the equivalent of a re-bore and this can be done at any age as long as the person is not too unwell. In their own right, however, TIAs can be treated by taking a small dose of soluble aspirin once a day (the aspirin makes the blood less sticky and less likely to form these small clots). There are other drugs available for people who cannot take aspirin for medical reasons. Unfortunately, repeated small stokes always cause some brain damage and if enough damage is done a form of dementia (multi-infarct dementia) can be produced.

Heart attack (myocardial infarction)

In this condition one or more of the blood vessels supplying the heart muscle become blocked and that piece of muscle is starved of oxygen and is damaged. In a young person this is accompanied by severe pain, usually described as 'crushing' and felt across the chest. The pain often goes down the left arm and up into the jaw. Similar pains lasting only a few minutes are called angina and are an indication that the blood vessels are furred up. Because this condition is so common, most younger people not only recognise the symptoms in others but also in themselves when it happens. This is not usually the case, however, with older people, especially the very old. They may have chest pain, i.e. a classic presentation, but most likely they will not. This is well recognised and referred to as the 'silent' heart attack. It is rarely silent in other ways though. It will commonly cause a collapse and often be associated with an acute confusional state. This is why doctors do a tracing of the heartbeat – an electrocardiogram (ECG) – in acute confusion. The tracing can sometimes look normal or have old changes present, so blood is usually taken to look for enzymes released by damaged muscle to help confirm the diagnosis.

Apart from confusion a heart attack can also cause shortness of breath due to poor heart pumping, leading to fluid on the lungs and abnormalities of the heart rate (either too slow, too fast or very irregular).

Severe diarrhoea and vomiting (gastro-enteritis)

All of us have experienced the unpleasantness of having diarrhoea (passing a very loose or liquid motion). It is usually a minor problem that goes away within a day or two. Sometimes it is more severe and is accompanied by lower abdominal pains. One needs to drink a lot of fluids. The condition may need the intervention of a doctor and occasionally drug therapy as well. However, such severe diarrhoea can make elderly people rapidly unwell. An older person can quickly get dehydrated (dry tongue, thirsty and eventually a state of collapse) and frequently become confused. This occurs twice as fast if the diarrhoea is accompanied by vomiting, as occurs in gastro-enteritis (and some other abdominal complaints including serious blockages). The actual cause of the diarrhoea may not be serious but its effects are. Cases where diarrhoea causes confusion need hospital admission. Many older people become incontinent of their motions when they get severe diarrhoea. This is distressing and difficult to manage at home. It was also always accepted as part of old age until a group of GPs were asked to question their younger patients about diarrhoea and incontinence. They found that at least 50 per cent of the younger people had also been incontinent during a bout of diarrhoea, but they had been too embarrassed to mention it to their doctor. The older patients were in fact no different.

In the very frail older person a frequent cause of diarrhoea and hence incontinence of liquid motions is in fact constipation. The hard motion in the back passage cannot get passed. The motions back up the bowel and finally liquid motion seep past the hard blockage. If this state of affairs is reached (faecal impaction) the hard motion has to be removed, after confirmation with an examination of the back passage by a nurse or doctor. An enema may be successful, but often the hard stool has to removed by manual evacuation. In the long term bowels must be kept regular. This is best done by a combination of as much exercise as is practicable, plenty of fluids and a varied high-fibre diet. Constipation on its own may make a person very uncomfortable and agitated but it is *not* a cause of confusion.

Chronic skin wounds

Leg ulcers

Leg ulcers are very common in older people. There are various types (venous, arterial and mixed), but the most common form is the venous ulcer, related to underlying venous disease and varicose veins. They can occur after minor injury to the ankle area and can enlarge rapidly. They are usually only moderately uncomfortable and severe pain should always require expert assessment to rule out arterial disease. The management of venous ulcers is to treat the surrounding skin with moisturisers (and treat any eczema with steroid cream) and compress them using a series of layers of bandages. This is done after the blood pressure in the foot has been measured to make sure that it is safe to compress the blood vessels. In this way most venous leg ulcers heal in about three to four months. The bandages are changed once or twice a week (depending on the amount of fluid leaking out – the exudate). Ulcers that do not heal in this period must be seen by an expert as there are many unusual causes of leg ulceration that can only be identified by a biopsy (the taking of a small piece of tissue under local anaesthetic).

A basic rule is that wounds heal best in a moist environment, hence all dressings are now prepared to stop the wound becoming dried out. Healing, however, can be a slow process and during the time that there is a raw area of tissue not covered by intact skin, infection is a possibility. There are many indications that infection (cellulitis) is occurring: the surrounding skin may get hot and red, there may be localised pain or the ulcer may begin to smell offensive. The wound may leak more fluid than normal, which may come through the bandages and be discoloured (green/yellow) or offensive. The infection can enter the bloodstream and cause an acute confusional state accompanied by general malaise and often feverishness. Skin infections like this need antibiotics and skilled nursing.

Pressure ulcers

These are variously known as pressure sores, bedsores or decubitus ulcers (Latin: *decumbere*, to lie down). Pressure ulcers are areas of dead skin and underlying tissues caused by pressure blocking the blood supply to an area of skin. They occur in older people who are immobile, frail, ill, and incapable of moving around unaided in bed or of shifting their weight in a chair. In almost all cases they are preventable by either regular turning or the use of special mattresses. It is not reasonable (or comfortable) for the patient to be turned every few hours and hence appropriate mattresses are the key factor in preventing this condition. About 10 per cent of all hospital admissions develop pressure ulcers – a scandalous figure. The condition can be painful, indeed life-threatening, and always increases the length of stay in hospital. It is also very expensive to manage. In addition, once present the wound is liable to infection, as with leg ulcers. The signs and symptoms are similar except that in many cases the wound is relatively insensitive and local pain may not be a major feature. Prevention is better than cure, but once the wound has occurred skilled management and advice is needed. If a pressure ulcer occurs in a hospital or nursing home setting, the patient and their carers should request an explanation. Pressure ulcers are an indication of poor quality care.

Sugar diabetes (diabetes mellitus)

The level of sugar in the blood is kept at a very precise level via insulin produced in the pancreas (a gland deep in the abdomen). In the condition known as sugar diabetes (diabetes mellitus) the body no longer controls the sugar level very well. There are two basic forms of the condition. In type 1 diabetes the problem is in insulin production and the person needs insulin injections to control the blood sugar. This usually starts when the patient is young, though some older people do develop the condition. Type 2 diabetes can also worsen in old age to a stage where insulin is needed. In type 2 diabetes (the milder form) the slightly raised blood sugar can often be controlled by diet (losing weight and avoiding very sugary things) or by taking tablets which lower blood sugar. Mild diabetes is more common as we age. If the blood sugar level does rise, symptoms include increased thirst, passing more urine than usual and a tendency to skin and urine infections. In elderly people high blood sugar can be caused by any infection present and may give rise to a state of confusion. When diabetes has to be controlled by tablets or insulin, care must be taken to ensure that the blood sugar level does not get too low, as this is a cause of confusion at any age but especially in older people.

If a person known to have diabetes becomes confused (especially if this is of rapid onset) then always give them a sugary drink or sugar in some form. It can be life saving when the blood sugar is very low (hypoglycaemia – which comes on quickly and is often accompanied by sweating) and will not cause harm if the blood sugar is in fact normal or raised.

*

The previous descriptions have concentrated on some of the more common medical conditions known to cause confusion in older people. It is also known that many non-medical occurrences can have a similar effect on the mental state.

Moving home

Many older people because of their frailty are encouraged to seek alternative accommodation. This usually means entry to sheltered housing or a residential or nursing home. Moving frail older people has risks however. There is an increased chance of severe illness (increased morbidity) including confusional states. There is also an increased chance of the person dying shortly after the move. These events are called the translocation effect. They have been studied closely and it seems that there are some precautions that can be taken to lessen the risks.

The premise on which these precautions are based is that no one should move unless they really have to. Some people have spent their whole life in one place and it is associated with family, events, emotions and a piece of them. There are many reasons why people do not cope in their own homes. Before embarking on a move, great care should be taken to ensure that the older person is not ill or that community and other services could not be mobilised a little more to keep the person in their own environment. If a move is needed, one only has to think of how traumatic moving can be when younger to appreciate how major a life event it is for the old. The elderly person may miss their home, neighbours and friends, and feel a sense of failure. The trauma can be minimised by ensuring that where possible the older person wants to move, i.e. it is a positive event. Forcing someone to move encourages complications. Many older people are frightened of the thought of so big a decision and need time and counselling by family and professionals to see the need and the help available for change. The person must then be involved as much as possible in the move. This means seeing and approving the new accommodation and deciding on such things as what personal belongings to take, etc. Special care must be taken when a move is contemplated for anyone who has any degree of confusion, as they are particularly prone to problems. The above plan is not, however, frequently the norm. Unfortunately, many moves occur at a time of crisis, resulting in a frightened individual being placed in a new environment by caring people, but for the wrong reasons.

Admission to/discharge from hospital

Admission to hospital and subsequent discharge is another traumatic time for older people. As described above, the actual move and change of environment is enough in itself to trigger off an episode of confusion. Add to this the reason for admission and hospitals can become dangerous places. Most people settle and recover and want to go home as soon as possible. A successful discharge depends, however, on many factors, the most important being communication. On admission, the team looking after the person needs as much information as possible, taking it from the patient concerned as well as relatives and other important sources (district nurses, home carers, etc.). In this way a picture is built up of the person in their home environment. This picture may reveal problems already present before admission and the reason for coming into hospital may itself throw up new problems. These need to be tackled in a systematic way with all the members of the multidisciplinary team using their expertise to get the person ready to return home. The patient needs to be fully involved, and in most cases a short home visit (a sort of trial run) is arranged to pinpoint or overcome any special areas of concern. A discharge date is then fixed, allowing patient, carers and services adequate time to prepare. Many hospitals use checklists to ensure that the correct type of ambulance has been booked and that such things as house keys are available. In this way most (but not all) of the dilemmas associated with discharge can be dealt with.

Discharge arrangements have gained a high priority in hospital procedures and have also been formalised in government legislation (see Chapter 9, page 153). This means that should something go wrong with the discharge procedure the area of fault is readily identified. Minor hiccups, though irritating, are probably best unchallenged. More serious errors should be brought to the attention of the ward manager, not only for the issue to be resolved and an apology given, but so that similar errors can be avoided in the future. Very serious problems are best followed up by a written letter of complaint, detailing the issues and sent to the hospital's customer relations department with a copy to the ward manager or consultant. This should ensure a prompt, detailed and effective reply.

Falls

Falls suffered by elderly people are the subject of numerous books. Suffice it to say that unless a good history concerning the circumstances surrounding the fall is available, showing that it was truly accidental, then a medical reason should be sought as to the cause. Accidental falls can nevertheless be extremely unpleasant. The degree of physical damage is often slight, but the shock to the system and to the person's confidence can be enormous. Not only can an acute confusional state be precipitated but the person may withdraw and not go out, using furniture to hold on to in the home and creating a dependency environment. Falls due to silent ill health are often accompanied by acute confusion. In the old and frail falls can be an indicator of brewing illness and have serious consequences. In some studies, many people who have fallen regularly have died shortly afterwards.

Falls are so common in old age that special 'falls clinics' have been established to help in diagnosis and management. The GP should be aware of the local clinics available.

Bereavement

The death of loved ones comes to us all. In old age it is perhaps more poignant to lose one's partner of a lifetime or friends who one knew at school. Perhaps most distressing is the loss of one's own children at a time when one was beginning to depend on them more and more. Grief knows no age barriers and is as intense at 80 as it is at 20. Bereavement can be another significant life event coming closely on the heels of many others at this time (loss of status, job, money and perhaps home and health). Most older people cope with bereavement naturally, but some, especially the very frail, may not. Confusion can occur. In most cases it is self-limiting and is helped if the natural grieving process can occur, for example by saying goodbye at a funeral service. Many carers feel that the older person should be spared the ordeal of the funeral, but in most cases it is a positive experience. There is a need to be present and contribute, to say farewell and begin the process of moving on to a different phase of life.

Failing eyesight and hearing

Failing vision and hearing are common symptoms in old age, so common that many people take them for granted as part of the ageing process. These two complaints should always be taken seriously and acted upon as soon as possible. There are numerous causes of both that are fully treatable or can at least be helped. Cataracts (opacities in the lens of the eye) are eminently treatable in most cases by surgical removal, even in the very old and frail. Glaucoma (failing vision due to increased pressure in the eye) needs to be diagnosed early to prevent further damage. Eye drops or surgery help preserve what sight is left.

Wax in the ears is the most common form of deafness and is easily treated. Deafness should be vigorously investigated and hearing aids supplied where necessary. Increasingly, hearing therapists are giving practical help and advice on the hearing disorders of older people. Sadly, a minority of elderly people do have significantly impaired vision and hearing. The two conditions occurring together is especially disabling. The person concerned may misinterpret vision and sound, and this renders them very prone to confusional episodes. These risks can be lessened by maximising their existing vision and hearing as much as possible. The person will usually relate very well to their familiar environment and carers, and within reason these should not be changed. Great problems occur when the person has to be moved or carers change. A lot of time has to be spent patiently re-orientating the client to any new surroundings, both environmental and human.

The management of acute confusional states

Before diagnosis and management can take place, the patient or carer has to recognise that something is wrong. This may be straightforward if the confusion is associated with markedly abnormal behaviour, with incontinence or other physical symptoms. It is less easy when the confusion is not severe and there are no other obvious complaints. If an older person becomes confused and this is picked up by carers, medical advice should always be sought. The sufferer themselves may be reluctant to see a doctor and carers may 'not want to bother the GP' but these feelings should be overcome because the sooner the correct diagnosis is made the better the outcome.

Once the cause is found, specific treatments can be given. In the most serious cases admission to hospital may be required. Common causes such as urinary tract infection usually respond very well to antibiotics. Confusion associated with slight strokes may take longer to respond. In addition to the specific treatment of the cause of the confusional state there are general measures that can be undertaken both at home or in hospital. The older person should be cared for in a calm environment. Loud noises (startling and frightening for anyone) should be avoided and the room should be well lit. This will stop the sufferer misinterpreting shadows, etc., which can provoke visual hallucinations. If very confused, the person should have a carer present. This will lessen the person's anxieties, and the carer will be able to cater to their needs (drinks, trips to the toilet) and ensure some degree of safety. If in hospital, the patient should be allocated the same nurse as often as is possible to avoid frequent face changes. A quiet, warm, well-lit room has a very calming effect on an agitated confused person. The drinking of plenty of fluids should be encouraged (water, tea and diluted cordials, *not* the superconcentrated sugary fizzy drinks guaranteed to make almost all older people have high blood sugar levels). The taking of full meals is less important for a few days.

Treatments will obviously take a few days to work, and during this time the elderly person may be quite agitated and distressed. Someone in this state must not be physically restrained unless they are about to harm themselves or others. If that is the case then minimal force should be used to keep them safe. Restraining encourages aggressive outbursts. A guiding hand and calm but firm voice works well, and distracting tactics are effective. Tip back chairs with restraining trays, cot sides and the tying down of limbs have no place in the management of acute confusion. If the person is in great danger of falling out of bed due to agitation, then the mattress should be placed on the floor, family and carers being fully informed as to the reason why. Boxing glove type mittens can be useful to help prevent drips, etc. being frequently removed. In hospital this type of situation needs a dedicated nurse to sit with the patient, 'specialing', until the agitation subsides.

It is often necessary to give some calming medication at the beginning of treatment when a person is excessively agitated. This is done to help keep the patient's dignity and to prevent them from harming themselves or others, as well as to avoid them becoming exhausted. Because elderly people are often on a large number of medications, hospital doctors will use small doses of the newer (atypical) anti-psychotics or benzodiazepines (for example, Diazepam). It is, however, recognised that benzodiazepines (like Diazepam or Lorazepam) can disinhibit patients further. In the first 24 hours of admission nurses should be vigilant for increased rather than decreased disturbances in behaviour.

In psychiatry of old age units there is a maxim for all medication: 'start low, go slow'. By which is meant that because *all* drugs have side effects, use the smallest or lowest dose possible and increase it (only if necessary) gradually. With the smallest but effective dose hopefully the patient can be made calmer without serious side effects. Too small a dose and the problems are worsened, as the agitated person is also sleepy and in danger of falling. Too large a dose and the person is 'knocked out' and misses fluids and meals, and the signs of the illness may be masked. These factors all contribute to the seriousness of the condition and the difficulties of management. One drug, Haloperidol (one of the original major tranquillisers), can be very effective and can be given in liquid, tablet or injection form. It does have side effects, but used in the smallest effective dose these are minimised. Its most troublesome side effect is to cause stiffness in the muscles and some rigidity similar to Parkinson's disease – this is called Parkinsonism. Any drugs given should be reviewed regularly and only given again if necessary. In most cases the dose can be lessened and the drug stopped once the other treatments begin working.

Acute confusional states are best managed by clinicians experienced in the treatment of older people, and the person should be reviewed by a psychiatrist of old age at an early stage.

Some of the most commonly used drugs for sedation have been used in the past as specific treatments for schizophrenia, for example Chlorpromazine or Clopixol. This should not be alarming since the drugs are used for their calming effects as well as their antipsychotic action.

Prompt recognition by carers and prompt diagnosis and action by GPs are the cornerstones of effective management and treatment for these rapidly developing states.

3

Chronic Confusion

Chronic confusion is defined as a confusional state that lasts longer than three months. In the previous chapter we looked at the causes of confusional states that usually do not last long. There are many causes of chronic, long-term confusion that can be reversed or greatly helped. The main differentiation is between these treatable causes and the irreversible conditions known as dementia. Chapter 4 will look at the main causes of dementia.

The significant point about chronic confusional states is that their causes may be reversible – no one should be diagnosed as having dementia until they have had a thorough screening for these treatable conditions. The diagnosis can often be very difficult and may need more than one period of assessment; for example, because of the time scale involved it is often difficult for carers to pinpoint when they started to feel concerned. The patient is not drifting in and out of awareness as in acute confusional states, and the problems vary with the underlying diagnosis. Memory loss and disorientation are common, but often the presentation is of someone failing to cope at home. The condition 'failure to cope' should always ring alarm bells.

The following is a list of conditions which will be discussed further.

- hypothyroidism
- Vitamin B12 and folic acid deficiency

- syphilis
- depression
- head injury and brain tumour (benign and malignant)
- normal pressure hydrocephalus
- Parkinson's disease and Cortical Lewy Body disease
- alcohol

Many of these conditions are entirely reversible. An accurate diagnosis of the confusion has marked implications for both the sufferer and the carers. The discussion below includes diagnosis and treatment.

Hypothyroidism

The thyroid gland in the neck produces the hormone thyroxine. The gland is the thermostat of the body and thyroxine is one of its regulators. It sets the level at which many of the body's processes run, including temperature. The gland often becomes less active in old age but it tends to do so slowly so that the effects only come on gradually. As the thyroxine level falls the body begins to slow down. The person becomes tired and slow, but as this happens over a long period of time many people put it down to old age. Gradually the symptoms worsen. People tend to put on weight, especially around the face, which gets very puffy. Body and mind start to slow down, including the bowels, so that constipation is a problem (another common problem, however, in old age). Even the pulse slows down as the body adjusts to a lower level of functioning. The person complains about the cold and feels they cannot get warm (indeed, their boiler is going out) and hair loss can occur from both the head and outer third of the eyebrows. If stressed (by cold weather) or illness the sufferer can lapse into a coma. As the disease progresses, mental faculties slow down with the rest of the body so that confusion in the latter stages is common. Because all of this happens over many months if not years, it can be very difficult for the patient or carers to notice these changes. Even the family doctor may miss it.

In its late stage the condition is readily diagnosable – the facial appearance, the husky gruff voice, slow pulse and slow relaxing tendon reflexes, as well as the symptoms of constipation and feeling the cold. A blood test confirms the diagnosis, and treatment is carried out by replacing the hormone thyroxine in tablet form. This has to be done extremely slowly at the beginning because the body has got used to a much slower pace. The dose can be increased gradually and everything returns completely to normal, including thoughts which may have become disjointed.

Because many of the symptoms and signs of this condition are rather non-specific (constipation and chronic confusion occur commonly together), the blood test to check the level of thyroxine and, more importantly, thyroid stimulating hormone (TSH) should be done on everyone with a chronic confusional state. TSH is a substance that increases in the blood stream as the thyroxine level falls. The thyroid replacement medication usually has to be taken for life. Hypothyroidism is especially common after the thyroid gland has been removed (thyroidectomy) because of over-activity when the person was younger. A thyroidectomy scar in a confused older person should always lead to the suspicion of hypothyroidism.

Vitamin B12 and folic acid deficiency

These two vitamin deficiencies will be discussed together because they often coexist and have similar symptoms. Vitamin B12 is found in meat (especially liver). It combines with a substance in the stomach and is then absorbed in the small bowel, where it enters the bloodstream. It is vital for healthy blood and it is important in the nervous system. Some older people fail to produce the 'intrinsic factor' in the stomach which vitamin B12 needs in order to be absorbed. People who have had part of their stomach removed (usually because of ulcers) may also fail to absorb the vitamin. The other name for this condition is pernicious anaemia because of its slow and debilitating onset. Folic acid is a vitamin found especially in fresh vegetables. It too is needed for blood making and for a healthy nervous system. Lack of this nutrient is usually due to a poor diet. Poor diets are probably caused 20 per cent by ignorance and 80 per cent by poverty.

The two deficiencies present in the same way. The person complains of tiredness and lethargy. If the nervous system is affected there may be complaints of abnormal sensation in the arms and especially the legs, with unsteadiness and a feeling that the person is walking on cotton wool. Walking may become difficult, confusion may gradually develop. The person looks pale and develops anaemia. They may have a pale lemon-coloured tinge to their skin. A neurological examination will often reveal abnormalities (in balance and sensation) and blood tests confirm anaemia with macro-cytosis (unusually big red cells). Confusion is reported late in the condition. These symptoms and signs lead the doctor to consider vitamin B12 or folic acid deficiency as the diag-nosis and to carry out the specific blood tests. Vitamin B12 can be measured in the blood, but as there are numerous causes for its deficiency other more sophisticated tests may have to be done as well. The folic acid content of red blood cells is the best blood test for folic acid deficiency, and this is routinely performed.

Until recently it was thought that vitamin B12 could not be given by mouth as the stomach acid destroys it, and the treatment generally continues to be by injections of the vitamin. These are usually then given every three months for life. Recent work, however, indicates that with special forms of oral vitamin B12 enough can be absorbed. Folic acid deficiency is easily treated by giving the vitamin in tablet form. Higher doses are given at the start of treatment and are then lowered to a maintenance dose, with improvements to the diet where necessary.

The longer these conditions have been present, the less likely it is that all the neurological complications will be reversed. The anaemia usually improves well, but where chronic confusion is established there are few reported cases of the mental state returning completely to normal.

Syphilis

Syphilis is a venereal disease that is usually sexually trans-mitted. The stage of the disease that can cause mental changes such as confusion occurs many years (often 20 or more) after the initial infection. The first stages may have been missed (painless lesions on the genitals and then rash-es) or the infection may have been inadequately treated at that time. Any person with a chronic confusional state must have a blood test for syphilis. The results can be complicated if inadequate treatment has occurred. Partially positive tests can occur and the specialist departments (Genito-Urinary Medicine – GUM) can offer advice. Often it is important to test the spinal fluid for syphilis by doing a lumbar puncture. This usually involves the person having a brain scan (CT scan) to make sure it is safe to do the test. The blood test can appear positive, but the spinal fluid tests negative, indi-cating that the infection is not causing the patient's states of confusion. It can be very difficult to do a lumbar puncture in some older people and then treatment is carried out according to the blood tests.

Treatment can be by daily penicillin injections for a few weeks or by oral antibiotics for a longer period. Unfortunately, the person may have passed on the infection to their spouse or children and so positive cases need to be referred to the specialist GUM department. Their skilled councillors can interview relatives and explain the need for further tests on them. The sooner the infection is treated the better the results. By the time the disease has caused a confusional state, complete recovery of full mental faculties is unlikely.

Depression

Depression in older people has also been called pseudo-dementia, i.e. false dementia. This is because the symptoms and signs of depression can be very difficult to distinguish from those of some of the dementing illnesses. Depression is common in old age and older people have the highest rate of successful suicide attempts. Depression frequently accompanies physical ill health and, as we have seen before, old age is also a time of loss, making coping with the burdens of everyday life that bit more difficult.

All of us have days when we feel sad, but for most of us the mood passes. A problem occurs when this melancholic outlook on life persists and begins to intrude into the person's daily activities. Common feelings in depressed people are of worthlessness and a hopelessness for the future. Sleep becomes disordered and there is early morning waking with an inability to get back to sleep and a subsequent feeling of a poor night's rest. Gloomy thoughts intrude and ideas of suicide begin to form. The person may worry about their general health and consult their doctor about many trivial complaints (hypochondriasis) or they may begin to feel that their body is rotten and that they are decomposing internally. Many slow down and lose the will to do anything, even speak. The person may refuse to eat and drink, and thus put their life in danger (this is called psychomotor retardation).

The condition gets muddled with dementia because by the time the person sees a doctor it may not be possible to obtain a thorough history. Various questions are asked to try to get an impression of orientation and memory and establish a diagnosis. Often the person does not answer and so scores badly. Given sufficient time and patience, correct answers can often be obtained, differentiating the condition from dementia, but in severe depression diagnosis is frequently difficult. Some people have a long history of depression, others have their first attack in old age. Making the diagnosis is the first step, and the sooner the better. Most people with depression do go to their GP but often do not complain of feeling low. The astute GP will realise that something is wrong and begin to ask the right questions, but still the diagnosis is often missed. In difficult cases the person should be referred to an old age psychiatrist. There is still great stigma attached to psychiatric disease, which is odd considering that a significant number of the population will suffer from a mental health problem during their lifetime. As psychiatric units cease to be housed in vast institutions and become part of the general hospital or community facilities, and as education continues, hopefully this prejudice will fade. There has been a tendency for GPs to consider the diagnosis of depression, but be reluctant to prescribe anti-depressants for this older age group. Fortunately, this is changing. Good clinical practice is to use the newer antidepressant drugs, as soon as the diagnosis is made.

In a few, the depressive illness will be part of a reaction to bereavement or disability or other stressful life events. It can herald cancer. Most of these cases will be monitored by the GP and the psychiatrist, and counselling may be beneficial. In the other cases antidepressant drugs are needed as well as support networks (day hospital, self-help groups, counselling, community psychiatric nurse). Drugs are very effective and have far fewer side effects than was once the case. One common group are called Selective Serotonin Re-uptake Inhibitors (SSRIs). Most courses of treatment are given via the GP or on an outpatient basis. Sometimes, however, the condition of the person is so severe that treatment has to be started on an inpatient basis. Medication may not be the only treatment, and in severe cases or where the condition is life threatening electro-convulsive therapy (ECT) is used. Many people who do not understand this form of therapy or who have never seen it given in a controlled modern setting are opposed to it. It is an effective, safe and necessary form of therapy in severe depression. A light anaesthetic is given and one electrode placed on the side of the head gives a minor shock, often just enough to cause a slight twitch. The side effects can include memory loss for a few days up to six months after the actual ECT in some people. There is, however, no permanent damage. Both drug treatments and ECT are usually given voluntarily. Occasionally, however, the depression is so severe that the person does not recognise that they are seriously ill and they have to be admitted to hospital under one of the Sections of the Mental Health Act (see Chapter 8, page 135).

Recovery from depression using ECT can be extraordinary, but some people will relapse and may need further courses of ECT or drug treatment. Because depression is common and treatable, great lengths must be taken to ensure that no one is labelled as 'demented' when in fact they are suffering from depression. Occasionally, the two conditions coexist. As the depression is treated the dementia does not go away but is usually noted to be less severe.

Head injury

A confusional state following a head injury must always be taken seriously, and it is important to note that confusion can occur some time after the event. Head trauma can be dangerous because the injury may have caused bleeding on the surface of the brain under the bone (subdural or extradural haematoma – or blood clot). If the bleeding is severe the confusion will become apparent at the time, the person becoming rapidly unwell and either losing consciousness or looking as if they have had a stroke. Bleeding can be less severe at the time of injury and the person appears to recover from the head injury, only to become unwell later. The symptoms can vary from bouts of drowsiness (fluctuating consciousness) to episodic or chronic confusional states. The collection of blood on the brain is best shown up using a CT scan (computerised tomography), where a computer generates from serial pictures 'slice' views of the brain – an image which is anatomically precise. If the collection of blood is large it can be drained by a neurosurgical operation. Recovery can be complete, but it does depend on the degree of damage sustained.

Brain tumour

It is rare for older people with a brain tumour to present solely with a slowly progressive confusional state. Usually the confusion is accompanied by other symptoms and signs such as headache, weakness of the limbs (usually on one side only) and falls. Brain tumours are ultimately diagnosed in the same way as a collection of blood, by using a CT or similar scan. Unfortunately, most brain tumours in older people are malignant and are secondary deposits (metastases) from a main tumour growing elsewhere in the body. Primary brain tumours of many types do occur but the prognosis for all of them is quite poor. Most tumours respond temporarily to high dose steroids or radiotherapy, both of which shrink the swelling around the tumour and to some extent the tumour itself to stop it pressing on other vital brain structures. The type of tumour and especially its rate of growth affect the prognosis, but in most cases it is not good. At an early stage the patient and the family need to be put in contact with the support systems available, such as palliative care teams, for example Macmillan nurses.

Benign (non-malignant) brain tumours, such as meningioma, are rare. When they are detected as part of a screening procedure for chronic confusion they can be removed, depending on their size, position and on the physical state of the person concerned.

Brainscans

There is debate as to whether all cases of chronic confusion should have some form of brain scan (CT scan – see page 117 – or the more recently developed MRI – magnetic resonance imaging). When all cases of chronic confusion are screened in this way the pick-up rate for brain tumours, collections of blood and other rare conditions is low. But the cost of failed diagnosis is very high to the individual and also, in financial terms, to the health service. Accurate diagnosis should not be a lottery. The outcome in terms of type of care, prognosis and impact on carers between a diagnosis of dementia and that of brain secondaries is very different indeed. Current resources are rationed, but people with chronic confusion are increasingly being screened by CT scan. Until this procedure is universal, however, it remains very important to scan those people where the suspicion of a treatable or relievable cause is high and to encourage discussion between GP, elderly care physician, psychiatrist of old age and neurologist at every opportunity.

Normal pressure hydrocephalus

This rare condition is included because it can present with a chronic confusional state and if diagnosed early it can be treated with neurosurgery. Normal pressure hydrocephalus is an enlargement of the chambers inside the brain which contain fluid. It can occur following different forms of brain injury, such as stroke, or it can develop on its own. The consequences are threefold: the person develops difficulty in walking (ataxia), becomes incontinent of faeces (and can also be incontinent of urine) and develops confusion (usually described as loss of short-term memory). These three problems are often present together in people with advanced dementia, hence the importance of recognising the problem early. The diagnosis is made on the history, examination and findings on the CT scan, as well as some other tests.

If the condition is discovered early, the potential for recovery is good. A shunt (a long tube) is passed from the chambers in the brain (ventricles) to the blood stream or down into the body cavity in the abdomen. In this way the build-up of cerebrospinal fluid (CSF) is diverted and the chambers start to revert to their normal size. In the past the diagnosis has been made late and the results of surgery have not been good, with little recovery in mental function and the complications of the surgery to contend with. Early intervention can produce dramatic improvement and full reversal of symptoms.

Parkinson's disease

This is a condition whose name is very familiar but of which clinical details are less well known. It was first described by James Parkinson in the 19th century and his description of the first six cases has never been bettered.

Parkinson worked as a doctor in Shoreditch in the East End of London and whilst out in the local market he saw two men, both of whom were running. The one in front was upright and the one behind severely stooped and only kept from falling by the front man's hand under his chin. He watched them run through the market area daily and gradually got to know them. They were brothers. As the one became more bent over he could only stagger forwards, getting faster and faster, and would fall over without his brother's help. Parkinson made a study of the stooped brother and over the years found five other cases that he wrote up for his medical report, describing them as having the 'shaking palsy'. His detailed assessment of the condition, later to be named after him, missed very few symptoms and signs. Parkinson did state, however, that he thought in this condition the intellect was spared. This is now being questioned (see Cortical Lewy Body disease, page 55).

Parkinson's disease is one of the most common neurological disorders of older people. It has many special features. One is the tremor of the fingers and hand. This usually starts on one side and is very rhythmical; the fingers are said to resemble someone who is 'pill rolling'. There is difficulty in starting a movement so that getting out of a chair or bed can be very difficult. The muscles become more stiff and rigid so that movements are slow and the face becomes blank and staring as the facial muscles become affected. All movements become disordered and the person tends to fall easily because they cannot balance well. As the disease progresses they tend to stoop forwards and hence fall forwards. To try and prevent themselves overbalancing the person takes little fast steps and may find themselves at a trot. The natural arm swing during walking gradually declines so that the arms hang by the side. Even the muscles in the gullet can be affected, making swallowing difficult. The skin can become very greasy, with a tendency to spots and blemishes, and bladder control is affected, causing a feeling of extreme urgency to pass urine and often incontinence. Some of these features may not occur at all in some people when the disease is very mild, for others the symptoms and signs described come on over a matter of years, causing increasingly severe disability. All aspects of daily life can be affected, even down to handwriting, so that letter and cheque signing becomes impossible and buttons and laces are something to avoid.

Depression is very common in this condition; it is both caused by and connected to the disease. The expressionless face and slow, often whispered, speech can lead people to think that the person behind the 'mask' must be addressed as a child. Chronic confusion can be a feature of the condition, but most sufferers' minds are alert, trapped in a body that won't do what they want it to. The greasy skin, tendency to drool at the mouth, urge incontinence and immobility add to the distress and misery. Depression should always be looked for because it is treatable and can make a big difference to the quality of life of the person with Parkinson's disease.

Unfortunately, as the disease progresses, there is a tendency for the sufferer to become confused. At the end stages the condition appears somewhat like Alzheimer's disease, and the same changes are found in the brain. This advanced form of Parkinson's is known as Cortical Lewy Body disease (see opposite for more information). For many, intellectual impairment occurs at the same time that the disease stops being sensitive to drug therapy and this coincidence is often a terminal event. For some, however, mental deterioration appears to occur earlier, and this makes management of their illness especially difficult.

The basic cause of Parkinson's disease is not known. We do know that all the movement problems and the tremors are secondary to the loss of a chemical in one part of the brain. This chemical is used to transmit messages to the nerves and then the muscle cells. The chemical is called dopamine and is made and stored in a tiny part of the brain called the substantia nigra. It is not known what causes the chemical to disappear, but symptoms do not appear until at least 90 per cent of it has gone, and this probably takes many years. A picture very similar to Parkinson's disease can be caused by numerous small strokes, drugs and even Alzheimer's disease – this condition is called Parkinsonism.

The treatment of Parkinson's disease involves many different factors. Initially a lot of improvement can be gained from physiotherapy. As the disease progresses, however, it is usual for drug therapy to be used. The most commonly used drug is levodopa (contained in Sinemet and Madopar). This treatment aims to put back the missing chemical. It has revolutionised the treatment of the condition but it does not cure it. It helps control the symptoms but the disease is usually continuing to progress silently. It is government advice that patients with Parkinson's disease should be referred to specialist centres (usually led by neurologists), where treatment options can be considered. However, confusional states can be a side effect of most of the drugs used to treat Parkinson's, especially if high doses are used. If a person with Parkinson's disease develops confusion, the drugs they are on must always be considered as the possible cause.

There is no doubt that as sufferers live longer they are becoming resistant to physiotherapy and drug treatment alone and they are becoming very disabled. There have been exciting research treatments, including the implantation of foetal brain cells into the depleted area and electronic devices to minimise tremors. Early results indicate very mixed results. It is always important to keep abreast of the latest developments, and this is best done through membership of the Parkinson's Disease Society and via the Internet (see Appendix 2 for Useful Information). Research centres sometimes recruit patients into various clinical trials where, provided the patient meets the requirements and is fully agreeable with the regime, they may benefit greatly from close scrutiny during the trial.

Cortical Lewy Body disease

It has been recognised for many years that people with Parkinson's disease may go on to develop a chronic confusional state. There has been much debate as to whether this was in fact Alzheimer's disease. Recently, improved techniques for looking at brain tissue under the microscope have shown the probable cause of Parkinson's disease to be a fall in the amount of the chemical dopamine produced. It is the balance between dopamine and the other chemical transmitters that is the basis for normal movement. In addition, small collections of protein appear within the brain cells. These are known as Lewy bodies. Until recently Lewy bodies have only been found in the same area as the dopamine producing cells, the brain stem. They are thought to be made up of various pieces of the cells' component parts coming together as the cell dies. New staining techniques have now shown them to be present throughout the brain in those patients with the confusion associated with Parkinson's disease. Researchers in the field have called this form of chronic confusion Cortical Lewy Body disease (CLBD). It represents the third most common form of dementia. It appears that the disease can start as Parkinson's disease and develop into dementia or it may start as a chronic confusional state which is later diagnosed as dementia, with Parkinsonian features developing later.

The condition is separate from Alzheimer's disease but has some similar features. The dementia CLBD affects memory, language, praxis (complicated actions) and gnosis (recognition of what things are) just the same as in Alzheimer's disease. There do appear to be some differences however. The cognitive impairment (all the brain functions such as memory) in Cortical Lewy Body disease has a fluctuating course, which is not so in Alzheimer's disease. There are some prominent features including a marked tendency to visual and auditory hallucinations, delusions and some aggression and depression.

The discovery of this new condition may have far-reaching consequences for the diagnosis of chronic confusional states. Many people with a diagnosis of 'dementia' go on to develop features of Parkinson's disease, including stiffness and some tremor. This has been put down to Parkinsonism. It may be that we will need to re-evaluate these cases and consider a diagnosis of Cortical Lewy Body disease.

Alcohol

As many people have learnt to their cost, the effects of acute alcohol consumption can be both seen and felt. Older people are no different in this, though their tolerance of alcohol may diminish. Initial feelings of well-being give way to increasing loss of social inhibitions, unsteadiness, slurred speech and difficulty concentrating, then to aggressive tendencies, nausea and vomiting, and finally to falls and unconsciousness. All of the above can occur even faster if alcohol is mixed with medication. Thus alcohol abuse should be considered in all cases of acute and chronic confusional states.

Some elderly people have carried their alcohol abuse along with them for years, though they are probably in a minority, for the effects of severe alcohol abuse are not compatible with a long life. These chronic abusers may show the effects of alcohol on every body organ. The liver may be cirrhotic (severely scarred and fibrotic), and after bouts of heavy drinking the skin may become yellow (due to a form of hepatitis – inflammation of the liver). General nutrition is often poor and the person can look malnourished – thin with a poor complexion, bad teeth and skin, a tendency to bruise easily and susceptibility to chest infections. This poor nutrition can be general or more specific if certain vitamins are missing. Alcohol abusers can be deficient in the vitamin thiamine and consequently present with falls due to an inability to walk properly (ataxia – not the acute effects of alcohol), eye problems and an acute confusional state – Korsakoff's psychosis. A very rare condition called Wernicke's encephalopathy is the irreversible result of not treating this condition.

If the supply of alcohol is suddenly withdrawn from a chronic abuser (for example on admission to hospital or residential or nursing care) then delirium tremens (DTs) can occur. This is a very dangerous condition, indicated by a craving for alcohol followed by confusion accompanied by hallucinations. The condition can be fatal, especially in the more frail older abuser. The long-term effects of alcohol on the brain are equally as bad. Alcohol is a well-recognised cause of chronic confusion or dementia. Memory loss is accompanied by a deterioration in the personality. The emotional trauma to family and carer is very great indeed – they have to cope with a dementing person who is made regularly worse by bouts of heavy drinking and who is usually very difficult to engage in long-term treatment.

Some people only turn to alcohol late in life. It may be possible to find a precipitating cause such as bereavement, depression or a chronic painful medical condition. These people usually present with frequent falls or frequent bouts of confusion that disappear after 24 hours in hospital. They have not been drinking long enough for the long-term physical signs to show, and their bodies are not dependent on alcohol so they rarely get DTs. Alcohol may be smelt on the breath or found in the blood in someone who is unconscious. More commonly, empty bottles are found in the bedside cabinet during an assessment visit to an old lady who is falling over a lot.

Long-term dependence on alcohol is as hard to treat in older people as it is in younger age groups. A commitment to abstain from alcohol has to be present. There are many organisations that can help, but few centres for rehabilitation of alcohol abusers will consider older people. The late onset drinker has a better prognosis, for it may be possible to identify the cause of the drinking and treat it. A few people appear to develop a drinking habit detrimental to their health after they have become confused with a dementing illness such as Alzheimer's disease and these few can be particularly difficult to help.

4
The Common Dementias

Alzheimer's disease was first described in 1907 by Alois Alzheimer. He performed a microscopic examination of the brain of a woman aged 51 who had died of 'dementia'. She would now be classified as having 'pre-senile' dementia. The term dementia at that time was also associated with schizophrenia, because younger people (in their 20s and 30s) with an equally tragic disease had some features that resembled older people with 'senility'. Today, of course, we have delineated many different types of mental illness. What Alzheimer described anatomically – changes in cell structure and deposits of a substance known as amyloid with an aluminium core – remains valid. He also found that a large proportion of the cells were tangled, and we now know that certain chemicals necessary for transmission of information within specific brain areas are diminished or absent completely. Memory and other functions are dependent upon chemical 'messengers' which are released from the ends of nerve cells within the brain. Acetylcholine (Ach) is now thought to be the main chemical messenger that is altered, although other transmitters are also affected. These physical changes are at the root of the problems that Alzheimer's dementia causes.

You should be aware from the outset that ultimately all the dementias, whilst having particular symptoms that cluster and being defined as a syndrome, are initially always a medical diagnosis (what the doctors think is the cause), which is only confirmed if the patient is examined at post mortem. Some centres advocate brain biopsy to clarify the diagnosis, particularly in younger adults, but even this is not always conclusive. The clinical picture is usually apparent to the experienced clinician, and with advanced psychological testing, neuroimaging techniques (brainscans) and a good history one can be 80 per cent sure of an accurate diagnosis. The course of the illness can also be roughly predicted, based on age at onset and any family history of the disease. The diagnosis can be complicated, however, by other co-existing physical illness, and frequently a superimposed 'acute confusional state' due to infection, etc. makes the whole picture seem much worse than would the dementia taken alone.

The term 'Alzheimer's disease'

Alzheimer's disease (AD) is a confusing term. It has become synonymous with other quite different pathological processes which are degenerative (destructive) brain diseases, but with different causes and outcomes. No one has yet fully pieced together the complex genetic and environmental factors that play a part in causing Alzheimer's disease, although it is by far the most common cause for referral among the dementias (50–70 per cent), with the two other major conditions being vascular dementia (caused by strokes) and dementia of the Lewy Body type (seen in Parkinson's disease). Post mortem studies have shown that not only are these three types the most common causes of dementia but that they also frequently occur together, for example 20–30 per cent of AD sufferers also have vascular dementia. Similarly, around 15–30 per cent of AD patients show Lewy Body pathology. This can make for a confusing medical picture and complicates treatment.

If one does not know anyone with dementia, the picture that one imagines can be bewildering and frightening. The onset is usually insidious and slow and may not be noticed for some time, often for as long as two or more years. Occasionally progress of the illness can be rapid. In this case the patient develops the disease earlier in life – so-called 'pre-senile dementia'. Characteristically the patient becomes withdrawn and less capable, and is not able to remember recent events. Odd and uncharacteristic behaviours occur. Sometimes this state is confused with depression, which can be an early accompaniment of dementia, and therefore should be treated. Nevertheless, there are some well-recognised 'operational criteria' (pointers to the condition and its diagnosis) both in Europe and in the United States that outline the clinical features of the dementias. These are known respectively as *The International Classification of Diseases 10th Edition (Chapter V – F00-F09)*, abbreviated to ICD 10, and *The Diagnostic and Statistical Manual 4th Edition* (DSM IV). It is as well to have heard of these criteria, since they are often quoted to relatives questioning the diagnosis, given what has been said above about uncertainty. These criteria have been shown over the years to be only 10–15 per cent inaccurate in their predictive value – that is to say, a diagnosis made using them is right more than 80 per cent of the time.

Description of the clinical picture

The word 'dementia' implies global deterioration in an individual's mental faculties (memory, reasoning, judgement, language) which occurs in the presence of brain disease (not just Alzheimer's) and is progressive and chronic in nature. It is a descriptive term and refers only to a syndrome and not to a specific disease. ICD 10 gives the following definition (WHO 1987):

Dementia is a syndrome due to disease of the brain . . . of a chronic or progressive nature, in which there is impairment of multiple higher cortical functions, including memory, thinking, orientation, comprehension, calculation, learning capacity, language and judgement. Consciousness is not clouded. The cognitive impairments are commonly accompanied, and occasionally preceded by deterioration in emotional control, social behaviour or motivation. This syndrome occurs in Alzheimer's disease, cerebrovascular disease, and in other conditions primarily or secondarily affecting the brain.

But what is it, Doctor?

Before we can start to think about a definitive diagnosis, we should look at how psychiatrists, neurologists and elderly care physicians begin to assess what the problem is and piece together a picture of what is happening to someone who presents with 'memory loss' or some other indicator of dementia. Initially the doctor, who may have considerable experience, will take a long history and perform a physical and mental examination. The doctor will be reluctant to confirm a diagnosis until all the tests have been done. Having collected all the data they will then be in a position to give the patient and relatives a likely diagnosis. The process is not overlong, but for the patient it can seem daunting and complicated, which it is. The whole subject of referral is discussed in Chapter 5, and assessment and treatment in Chapters 6 and 7.

Alzheimer's disease

When a person develops Alzheimer's disease, it often takes a long time for close relatives and carers to notice that anything is wrong. It is only when certain indications are pointed out that they can pinpoint the time when the dementia first showed itself. This is because a person has to lose a considerable amount of their 'working' brain before symptoms develop, possibly as many as 80 per cent of their cells. The problems occur late because the brain has cleverly adapted to the losses of brain areas. It is useful to think of the condition having three phases:

mild → moderate → severe

The progression is not entirely a linear one (i.e. a gradual decline). A small group of patients do have a very rapid downward course, with death occurring within a few years. For most, however, the course is quite slow, especially if the person is well cared for in a social atmosphere where they are mentally and physically stimulated, and any other medical problems are tackled early and effectively. Many people with Alzheimer's disease die of something else, such as heart attack or stroke, bearing in mind that Alzheimer's disease is now thought of as a multi-system organ failure in its end stage. Previously we might have called this 'old age'.

Alzheimer's is much more than memory loss, it affects all the parts of the brain that make us individual and allow us to relate and respond appropriately to other people. This is why carers find it so distressing, and the patient in the early stages is often very fearful and highly defensive against admitting they have a problem. This can make referral difficult, but ultimately early referral is the best course for patient and carer, since early treatment has been shown to slow and even stabilise the disease, allowing adjustment to the problem and appropriate home care to be put in place. Such help can keep the patient at home for much longer, helping to relieve care-givers' stress and delaying institutional care in whatever setting. Even in the very late stages a sufferer is able to express certain personality traits and respond to kindness and gentleness.

Is it genetic in origin?

It is still unclear whether the origins of Alzheimer's disease are genetic. A complex interplay of factors seems to be involved in the development of Alzheimer's disease and the other dementias. It is known, however, that first degree (father, mother, brother, sister) relatives of AD patients are three times more likely to develop the condition compared to non-affected families in the population. Nevertheless, most cases are sporadic, that is arising from 'nowhere', seemingly out of the blue. Patients with Down's syndrome (who have an extra copy of chromosome 21) have a higher risk of developing AD, which has led to research into specific genetic markers and what have been termed 'specific pathogenic loci'. There is more evidence for genetic causation in early onset Alzheimer's disease, with mutations on chromosomes 21 and 14 producing protein abnormalities.

The genetics are complicated but evolving rapidly and are the target of newer trial treatments using antibodies (the bodies own immune defence system) to specific proteins in the brain. There is a strong association with a gene on chromosome 19 that makes a specific protein and late onset Alzheimer's disease. Around 40 per cent of AD patients, however, do not possess the specific gene that makes the substance called apolipoprotein E found in plaques and tangles in the brains of sufferers, so its presence alone is neither necessary nor sufficient for the development of the disease.

Genetic testing is *not* at present advised or available outside research centres, where questions of ethics are still being debated. Other possible risk factors for AD include old age, infections, autoimmune conditions, head injury, aluminium, previous history of depression, advanced age of mother at birth and thyroid disease. None alone seems to be able to account for the development of this very complex pathology. Recently, in the light of publicity of new Variant Creutzfelt Jacob disease (nVCJD) or 'mad cow disease', some attention has focussed on slow viruses, but the pathology seen is very different from that of Alzheimer's disease.

Common problems found in Alzheimer's disease

It has recently been discovered by research at The National Hospital for Nervous Diseases, in London, that some first degree relatives of patients with a strong family history of Alzheimer's disease, if tested around the age of 50, have memory problems that they don't even notice. Psychologists have now developed very specific techniques and batteries of tests for memory loss that can detect very early changes in brain functioning. This is very good news if you want to treat patients as early as possible, given a suspicion that they may develop AD in the future. Memory loss occurs in *all* cases of AD, but it can be difficult to detect as people cover it up very well. It is the recent memories which go first, and only much later in severe disease does the long-term memory become affected. In 1974 a test called the Folstein Mini Mental State Examination was developed to screen patients not only for memory loss but also for other features of dementia. The test consists of 30 questions (see page 66) and is a good way to screen patients at an initial visit, but it is by no means totally accurate. Many people still test memory with the abbreviated mental test score, as follows:

- How old are you?
- What is your date of birth?
- What is the day today?
- What month are we in?
- What year is it?
- When was the First World War?
- What is the name of the Prime Minister?
- Where are you now?
- Remember an address, for example '24 West Register Street', and ask the person to repeat it after five minutes.
- Count backwards from 20 to one.

Mini Mental State Examination (Folstein et al)

Patient name _____

Date of birth _____ Date of test _____

SECTION	MAX POINTS	PATIENT SCORE
1 Orientation		
What is today's day/date/month/year/season?	5	
Where are we?		
Town or city/county/country/building/floor?	5	
2 Registration		
Name 3 common objects e.g. apple, chair, ball.		
Ask the patient to repeat all three.		
Repeat until all three are remembered.	3	
Number of trials needed ☐		
3 Attention & Calculation		
Start from 100 and keep subtracting 7.		
Stop after 5 answers: (93, 86, 79, 72, 65)		
OR		
Spell the word "WORLD" backwards (DLROW).	5	
4 Recall		
Repeat the three words I asked you to say earlier.	3	
5 Language		
Naming: Show a watch and pencil and ask the patient to name them.	2	
Repeating: Repeat the following "no ifs, ands, or buts".	1	
Reading: Show the sentence overleaf (Close Your Eyes). Read the sentence and do what it says.	1	
Write a short sentence on your own.	1	
Three stage command: Take a piece of paper in your right hand, fold it in half and place it on the floor.	3	
6 Construction		
Copy this diagram (see overleaf).	1	
TOTAL SCORE	30	

Examiner _____

Notes _____

Reference: Folstein MF *et al. J Psychiatr Res* 1975; **12**: 189–198

The Folstein Mini Mental State Examination

This is an easy test to perform, as long as the person is co-operative and has been asked nicely! The score out of ten should be 10/10, but lower scores should not be interpreted as dementia unless they are consistently given and produce the same results over time. The difficulty, as with most standardised tests, is that the results are dependent upon education and background. More refined testing is described in Chapter 6.

The other major areas that patients, or more frequently carers, may initially notice as problems, are:

- disorientation
- judgement
- personality
- speech
- activities of daily living
- sleep
- sexual behaviour
- risks to themselves or others
- incontinence
- restlessness and pacing

Disorientation

Disorientation involves not knowing where one is or the correct time, date, month, etc. It is so closely related to working memory that it is hardly surprising that it is an early feature of Alzheimer's disease. The information that is used least goes first. Gradually the person will become more muddled as to the correct month or day of the week. At this stage people are often 'well preserved' in other areas of daily life and are still managing shopping trips on the bus. However, gradually the patient becomes lost more frequently, first outside the home and then within it. Often a move or a holiday makes the disorientation more marked, and the patient becomes more fearful and anxious. Sameness and continuity of care is very important for the 'confused' individual. If environmental 'sameness' is maintained, then patterns of behaviour, including continence, eating, sleep, reading and attending to conversation or the television, can be maintained for longer.

The occupational therapist attached to a psychiatric or older persons medical unit has a crucial role in examining and resolving difficulties, both in the home and hospital settings. Their role is to test and maintain independence for as long as the disease allows, using prompts and aids to living. They are crucial to both assessment and follow up of dementia patients and can, with social services, delay or prevent institutional care, even without the newer treatment options. When 'wandering' becomes a difficulty, neighbours and the police often become concerned. What seems the most reasonable option to many families, however – moving the person nearer to them in order to supervise them more closely – often increases confusion and wandering behaviour. Almost inevitably, permanent institutional care follows, since there is often no alternative.

Repetition of phrases such as 'What time is it?' and 'What day is it?' by the patient can be addressed by tapping into residual new memory to sequence tasks that lead to the answer. Point to a clock or a calendar on a wall. These questions often drive carers to despair, but psychologists have found that after 20 repetitions patients simply stop asking and learn to check the clock or calendar. They do not remember why or how they came to know the process, but carers are relieved of the task of answering the questions over and over again. A *This Is Your Life* book can be used to remind a person who they are and how they relate to those around them. Labelling objects and rooms with bold lettering and hiding objects such as purses and keys can prevent a lot of hunting about! Always repeat visitors' names, since patients are often perplexed by the appearance of someone they think is their mother or father. It is my experience that arguing doesn't help much.

Judgement

Another difficulty for people with dementia is the eroding of complex, but hitherto ordinary things such as driving skills. Automatic functions seem to be preserved until the disease is well advanced, but at this point judgement or the lack of it becomes a problem. It is also challenging for anyone who is still working. These complex decisions are mediated by the frontal lobe of the brain, which is damaged early on in Alzheimer's disease along with the temporal lobe. Another area of the brain, the parietal lobe, organises motor skills like managing right and left and co-ordinating actions. The co-ordination of these various large brain centres may be faulty and may not correspond to what a patient thinks they can or cannot do. Conflict ensues, but protecting these vulnerable people whilst maintaining personal respect and autonomy should be at the core of all decisions. The legal problems and solutions for dementia patients are discussed in Chapter 8.

Personality

This is the crucial area for most families. Many Alzheimer's sufferers remain their old selves with some memory and orientation problems, but it is painful when a loved person becomes a coarsened shell of their former self, almost unrecognisable because of their actions and speech. In some sufferers underlying and predominant character traits come to the fore, such as anxiety or a tendency to verbal spitefulness. Personal hygiene may deteriorate, along with associated bathing habits. Carers notice stained clothes and a marked body odour, often made worse by the sufferer not recognising when they have finished toileting themselves. Carers may find this aspect of the condition particularly difficult, and it is often associated with strenuous denial by the patient that they have not washed or are other than perfectly clean. In a sense this is a part of judgement and also of failure to recognise and remember that things are amiss. Sexual inappropriateness is fortunately rare, although much feared if it has occurred once. It is not uncommon for arrests to be made for indecent exposure or undressing in public, but the police are fortunately much more knowledgeable about this problem now than they were in the past. Frontal lobe dementias are the focus of much study, and psychiatrists are grappling with how a pure frontal lobe 'picture' should be defined, for in this condition disinhibited behaviour is a prominent feature.

Speech

Speech is commonly affected in Alzheimer's disease. Initially word-finding difficulties occur, along with using the wrong word and sentences that are difficult to follow. Interpretation and receptive speech difficulties (understanding what we hear) follow, with conversation again difficult to follow. More complex functions such as metaphors in talking are omitted. As the disease progresses, understanding of simple commands is usually preserved, but frequent repetitions or nonsense sentences are formed which clearly have some meaning for the sufferer, but can only be interpreted by careful listening and familiarity with the person by the carer. Writing becomes more difficult, and reading, if tested, is also shown to be affected. The difficulty can be imagined if you think what it is like to try and understand a foreign language when several people are speaking at once. One feels cut off even if in full command of the social circumstances and with all brain functions intact. An interesting thing about native and learnt tongues is that it is the native (perhaps forgotten) tongue that again becomes the most useful to the person in moderate to severe Alzheimer's. These memory traces were laid down at the very beginning of the patient's life, and so it is not surprising that they revert to their first language.

In advanced disease the patient becomes mute and un-responsive to all but painful stimuli. It is at this point that carers have their hardest task. In hospital settings it can be extremely difficult – but rewarding – to communicate only with touch or visual cues. Speech is now mostly meaningless. The occasional verbal ejection or noise is usually nothing more than that, but touch or massage can calm the patient.

Activities of daily living (ADLs)

As all the main brain areas are affected in Alzheimer's disease, at some point difficulties with handling objects and understanding one's spatial (spacial) world occur. This is called 'dyspraxia'. Dressing dyspraxia is very common. It shows itself by the person putting on layers of clothes in the wrong order and back to front, etc. Buttons are frequently misaligned.

The holding of a knife and fork can be difficult, and a spoon can be substituted. If someone is losing weight it may be due to a failure to recognise that they have to eat, because they think they have eaten already or cannot remember how to prepare a simple meal. Meals on Wheels or bought in frozen and then microwaved foods are one solution, but malnutrition is not uncommon in the more unsupervised of sufferers. A limited or faddish diet consisting of chocolate, cheese and biscuits, tea and toast can be difficult for carers trying to ensure a balanced diet. Vitamin C in juices is a must, and most other nutrients can be found in wholemeal bread, fruit and vegetables.

If someone refuses to eat this should be investigated. There may be a simple reason, such as a denture problem or gum disease, or something more complex like a loss of taste sensations or a sense of difficulty in swallowing.

Sleep

Most people agree that as we age we need less sleep. However, some of us still need more than others. The past should be a rough guide to the future of our sleep patterns. In AD the amount of sleep we need may not change, but what alters is the rhythm and distribution of sleep throughout the day – the 'sleep-wake cycle' changes. People with AD tend to be awake more at night and sleep more during the day. In one sense this does not matter, but it does affect carers whose daily balance is thrown by sleepless nights and exhausted days.

It is best to avoid the use of medication unless it becomes absolutely necessary. Keeping the sufferer as active as possible throughout the day is often effective, so that they become tired by bedtime and exhaustion takes over. A little drink at night (brandy or sherry) after a warm drink and a bath may lead to less disturbed nights, so long as both mobility and continence are not a problem. Night sitting services are increasingly available, even if limited in the number of nights they can provide. This service, along with respite admission to residential or nursing homes, can provide a much-needed restorative break from caring. Arthritic pain can be helped by paracetamol, and night cramps by quinine from tonic water or quinine tablets.

There may be times when medication becomes invaluable, but the downside is that the brain is often affected and 'hang-over' effects are a problem, sometimes leading to increased disorientation and falls. Always consult your GP or local psychiatric service provider, who will have their preferred option and advise you.

Sexual behaviour

Although upsetting for carers these are often controllable, and dignity can be restored by simple devices such as fly-less trousers for both men and women, and impulse controlling medication and diverting activities. The problem may also be related to local urinary tract problems, so examination is usually advised. Whilst most professionals caring for dementia patients are aware that open masturbation and getting into the wrong bed may be problematic, in reality these are rare occurrences and are usually treated by separation and behavioural techniques – rarely medication. The main problem is in the home where a man (usually) has a resurgence of sexual interest in his wife that is unwanted on her part and difficult to fend off. If persistent, a temporary separation in respite care may give some space for reflection on what is a complicated dynamic, and the patient on returning home has often lost interest again.

Risks to themselves or others
Altered behaviours and judgement lead to exposure to risk. That carers feel they have failed a sufferer when something goes wrong is a recurring problem in practice, and the balance of risk-benefit must be individually tuned. It is never an easy topic to discuss, and there are rarely ideal solutions. Some risks (gas and fire) can be minimised, others (accidents and sudden illness) cannot. The right to remain at home, even though confused, is one that most of us would wish to see maintained, even with what some would view as unacceptable personal risks. It is a matter of temperament, carer involvement and team judgements.

Homes should be well lit, warm (automatic enclosed heating systems), secure (as far as possible without hindering escape in an emergency), with no open fires, gas, or hot surfaces. Double rails should be fitted to stairs and loose carpets and rugs removed. Remove clutter and unnecessary furniture so that walking sticks and zimmer frames do not catch and cause a fall. Alarm systems and a telephone are invaluable as well as warden alarms or those connected to the local police station. Ideally, medication should be locked away and the taking of it supervised. Lodge a spare set of keys with a known neighbour.

Increasingly, the problem of theft and other abuse is being recognised, especially when a person is known locally as confused or lives in sheltered accommodation where 24-

hour supervision is not the norm. Wandering is a particular and often defining moment for carers. It usually heralds higher or alternative levels of intervention, such as residential care. As a substitute for adequate supervision 'tagging' is unacceptable, although it may ultimately find its place among care options as diversity in living placements broadens. The greatest threat to personal safety is ultimately fire and falls, of which the latter take some time to overcome. Confidence may be eroded forever.

Incontinence

A very common problem accompanying dementia is urinary, and to a lesser extent faecal, incontinence. In most cases the person can be helped and, indeed, made continent again. However, there are many causes of incontinence and as many treatments, so it is important to ensure that the problem is diagnosed and the options evaluated thoroughly. For detailed information on incontinence, see Appendix 1, page 171.

Restlessness and pacing

This is a common behaviour exhibited by perplexed and aimless patients with dementia. It often makes them and their carer exhausted. It is extremely difficult to control without the help of medication; however, this has its own problems – for example, falls. Where possible both restlessness and pacing should be tolerated. Wandering areas in care homes can allow safe paths for distraction. Attempts to curb pacing can cause aggressive behaviour.

Problem behaviours

Surveys of distress amongst caregivers and patients give different inventories of causes. The main problem behaviours, averaged from eight studies, are listed below in order of most to least common. It should be noted that the least common 'difficult behaviour' occurs in one in four patients.

A patient might be expected to have at least one problem that is brought to medical or social work attention:

- verbal aggression and threats
- physical aggression and agitation
- restlessness
- sleep disturbances
- wandering
- apathy/withdrawal
- sexual disinhibition

Carers will need frequent breaks and access to informal and formal help in dealing with all the above in order to sustain kind and patient support and reassurance. Some psychiatrists would suggest 'rolling respite' for patients who are particularly demanding, whilst in other cases the family unit may be examined to detect poor coping strategies or situations in which behaviour becomes accentuated. In very advanced cases of dementia, very primitive and antisocial behaviours are manifested, causing considerable distress to carers, particularly spitting and biting, and also inappropriate defaecation and urination.

Inevitably carers request help with most of the above problems, and in our experience often want drugs to calm restlessness and improve outbursts of aggression. Respiridone (Respidal) and Olanzepine (Zyprexia) in tiny doses are often used. These drugs have advantages over the older major tranquillizers (neuroleptics) of not causing Parkinsonian symptoms (so-called extra-pyramidal side effects), which lead to falls and sometimes worsen confusion. Respiridone comes as a liquid and Olanzepine as a tablet that instantly fizzes on the tongue so that administration is easier for uncooperative patients. For their own safety and for that of others, patients are very occasionally admitted to hospital compulsorily under the Mental Health Act (see page 135) in order to treat them. This usually happens after several attempts have been made to encourage patients to take informal help when a worrying situation arises. Ultimately the MHA protects patient's rights as well as giving doctors power to treat someone who has lost their insight and cannot consent to treatment because of their illness.

Non-cognitive features

The effects of Alzheimer's disease are not just confined to cognitive features (also known as 'higher cortical functions') – memory, thinking, orientation, learning capacity, language and judgement. The disease also influences non-cognitive domains – behaviour, mood, thoughts and perceptions, sometimes leading to paranoid thinking and visual, auditory and olfactory hallucinations. These symptoms occur in up to 50 per cent of all patients with Alzheimer's-type dementia.

Delusions are ideas that are odd, strange and illogical but are fixed and not amenable to reason. Delusions fall into three common categories:

- delusions of theft
- delusions of suspicion
- systematised (complex) persecutory delusions

Alzheimer's disease also produces 'misidentification syndromes', where the patient can (cruelly it might seem to some) see a person as someone else. Four types of misidentification are commonly recognised:

- people in the house (family thought to be intruders)
- misidentification of a mirror image
- misidentification of television
- misidentification of people (for example, the patient takes her husband for her father)

Alzheimer's disease is also associated with depression in around 20 per cent of sufferers.

Vascular (multi-infarct) dementia

This disease is very different from Alzheimer's, although it is often confused with it. Alzheimer's disease accounts for more than 50 per cent of all referred cases of dementia and vascular (multi-infarct) dementia around 30 per cent. The remaining patients mostly have Lewy Body disease. A large proportion of patients have a mixture of both Alzheimer's and vascular dementia.

Vascular dementia (VD) is a result of repeated strokes. Sometimes the strokes are large enough to cause weakness of an arm or leg (or both), collapse, slurred speech and facial weakness (drooping). The brain is very dependent upon a constant supply of oxygen and nutrients, most importantly glucose. If this is interrupted, irreversible cell damage is caused in a matter of seconds. The extent of damage depends upon a number of factors, but essentially the larger the clot or burst blood vessel the greater the damage. The area affected is crucial to the symptoms seen, since not everyone with a paralysis due to a stroke has cognitive difficulties, although most people with this form of paralysis are depressed. If multiple insults of this type occur, it is because the main arteries supplying the brain are furred up and get blocked easily (atheroma or arteriosclerosis).

Because atheroma is not localised to the brain but generalised to the vessels of the body, vascular disease is easily diagnosed. The patient will have a history of atheroma-inducing disease (diabetes, hypertension and fat metabolism problems), will smoke and/or drink excessively and will often have had a fatty diet, although they may not be obese. They will usually have a history of blackouts, strokes and heart attacks, a fast or very irregular heart beat, breathlessness and pain on walking (intermittent claudication).

One-third of people recover from a major stroke almost completely, but another third have physical or mental impairment making them dependent upon others. A first stroke may go unnoticed or may affect memory and behaviour. These aspects usually recover, since the brain adapts, but the weakness of limbs and slurred speech often remain as a marker of the event. As the number of strokes increases (even in the presence of Asprin and anticoagulation medication such as Warfarin), the brain copes less and less well with each new insult. There is a 'step-wise deterioration', where the person never regains their former level of functioning.

Pathology

In vascular dementia there are large (visible to the naked eye) and small (microscopic) holes (lacunae) in the substance of the brain. The actual volume of brain lost is associated with the severity of cognitive impairment/dementia. Unlike in Alzheimer's there is *no* characteristic neurochemical imbalance. Brain scans are usually diagnostic.

Characteristics of the disease

Vascular dementia is the diagnosis of choice with someone who has an abrupt onset of signs and symptoms, affecting short- and longer-term memory, a relatively well-preserved personality and, most characteristic of all, 'sun-downing' or nocturnal confusion. All this is seen in the context of heart disease and the other risk factors listed above. Memory, as with Alzheimer's, is affected, but the problems are localised to one or two brain areas at first, and neuroimaging shows up multiple holes in the brain substance. It was Hachinski in 1974 who first proposed criteria for the 'probable' diagnosis of VD. More recent criteria take into account the results of scans.

Common problems

- gait (walking) disorders
- Parkinsonism
- emotional lability
- incontinence
- swallowing

A stroke has the effect of bringing our emotions closer to the surface; even though we try to control them, they can escape unwanted into the public gaze. Strokes lessen the amount of control one has so that patients laugh when they do not find anything funny (or disproportionately to the situation) or cry when they are not actually moved to do so. Such behaviour is called 'emotional incontinence' or 'lability' and is due to damage to the control centre in the frontal lobe of the brain. It appears that some of the older antidepressants (for example, Amitriptyline 10–25mg) in low dosage can control this. An antiepilepsy drug called Carbemazepine (100–200mg daily) is similarly useful.

Incontinence of urine (more often than faeces) can occur after a single stroke but is more common as multiple strokes lead to a confused state. Treatment of this problem (discussed in Appendix 1, page 171) may be more difficult because there is no underlying cause that can be sorted out. Although for reasons of dignity and resistance we try to avoid the incontinence pad and catheter, sometimes they are necessary and unavoidable for life to be bearable, for patient and carer.

Can we be sure?

As was previously said, with today's techniques we can be 80 per cent sure that we are dealing with a primary vascular pathology, but with up to 30 per cent of dementias having a mixed Alzheimer and vascular pathology at post mortem, there remain some patients who elude 'possible' (i.e. very likely) diagnoses.

Dementia with Lewy Bodies

There are no agreed criteria for diagnosing this illness, but it does have a very distinguishing hallmark: there are pronounced variations in attention and alertness, recurring visual hallucinations which are well formed in the sense that they are very graphic and 'real', and sudden onset of muscular rigidity as in Parkinson's disease. Patients often have multiple recent falls, transient 'blanks' or disturbances in consciousness, odd complex delusions and other hallucinations. If given certain drugs they react very badly. The degree to which a patient is affected is associated with the density, or number in a square centimetre, of Lewy bodies. Patients with Parkinson's disease can also develop this illness. See page 55 for more information on Lewy Body disease.

Other dementias

These are rare. But you might hear a doctor mention those due to normal pressure hydrocephalus, syphilis (making a comeback) or vitamin deficiencies (see page 44).

Age associated memory impairment

In 1986, in the USA, this term was devised to describe a particular *research* problem that doctors were trying to solve. The condition can be described as memory loss in healthy, elderly individuals in the later decades of life. At the end of the day what was being described was very early dementia, using a patient's subjective distress as the marker to identify affected individuals and very accurate psychological testing to confirm the diagnosis. The question is one of cut-off. All the subjects studied went on to develop dementia as more classically defined.

5

Where to Get Help

Formal and informal networks

Formal networks are those services supplied by various agencies. They are time and budget limited, and fairly inflexible but form a safety net for countless thousands of older people. Informal networks consist of family, friends, carers and neighbours. They provide services that are free, flexible in time and range, and usually provided with care and affection. Informal networks enable many older people to continue living in their own houses, aided where necessary by formal input.

'Formal networks' thus describes a whole raft of National Health Service, private sector and local authority provision that may also utilise voluntary services as part of the 'package' of care for the patient/client.

Health
- General Practitioner
- primary care services (community health services)
- mental health services
- secondary care services – acute hospital trusts
- NHS Direct

Local Authority
- social services (social workers, access to residential and nursing homes)
- housing services

Department for Work and Benefits
* benefits

Voluntary organisations
* Age Concern
* Help the Aged
* Alzheimer's Society

The National Health Service remains free at the point of entry and should provide a relatively seamless service throughout the contact with its various parts. Integration of health and social services budgets is proposed in the near future. This should make services less competitive with each other for money. The goal posts in the structure and organisation of the health service are changing rapidly, and have been since the 1980s, so it is impossible to predict what services will look like in 10 years time. What follows is a discussion of what is currently available.

For 'informal networks' read 'family, friends and neighbours'. These are the people who provide 24-hour help, often in emergencies, usually delivered with utmost attention to detail and love. Many carers carry on without help of any sort, and the vast majority are women. Local voluntary services and community schemes can come under this heading too, since they tend to work more flexibly. Being a carer can be stressful and can lead to unwanted feelings of resentment, and guilt about these feelings. There are several places to look for help, but we recommend an organisation like Carers National (details of which can be found in the phonebook or on their Internet website, www.carersnorth. demon.co.uk). Because caring can be intensive, many carers have lost social contacts and left jobs in order to do another full-time job that has no status or recognition beyond the home. Carers may also be embarrassed by the elderly person's odd behaviours and may have to control their own feelings of distaste. Such may be the situation that it can seem easier to stay at home rather than go anywhere public. Isolation can become a huge problem, as can depression and alcohol abuse. Sharing tasks with family and friends can ease the burden and make a social life outside the home possible, although guilt about 'leaving' someone is a constant anxiety carers voice. We would encourage involvement with community and charitable groups who can share their experiences with you and you with them. They are an invaluable source of friendship and support that allows most carers to continue the informal burden of caring for someone at home.

HEALTH

The General Practitioner

The General Practitioner is the focal point within primary care, and increasingly works in partnership with other GPs based in a health centre. These health centres then become the base for other primary healthcare workers and should be the main point of contact with most other agencies and a source of advice. Most GPs are self-employed and regulated by the health authority. After the days of fund holding (with GPs looking after their own budgets) came the Primary Care Groups and now Primary Care Trusts. GPs are becoming much more powerful commissioners of services than at any other time in the history of the NHS. They can now be involved in the planning and delivery of the local community health care services.

The government insists that anyone over 75 years old is offered a screening programme in which weight, hearing, eyesight and blood pressure are measured. This screening should also include some tests of cognition such as a basic screen for memory impairment. GPs are increasingly vigilant about the possibility of dementia, since it is so common. However, many delegate this screening role, and often practices do not follow up initial 'refusers' or 'non-attenders', so increasing the possibility of missing confused older people. The range of services GPs offer varies from excellent to poor, with some offering checks on levels of disability, evidence of depression, advice on abusive situations, etc. As consumers of services elderly people should be more critical of the service they are getting and shop around if not satisfied. The present Labour government seems determined to make the patient the centre of power in the health service.

Choosing a GP

The elderly patient and their carers should ask certain questions of their general practice. This may facilitate local standards to rise.

- Does the practice use an age/sex register? This enables the GP to be aware of the elderly population in the practice and plan the development of schemes for their benefit.
- Does the practice do its own house calls out of hours? Elderly people need continuity of care. The use of deputising services often means inappropriate measures being taken, and hand-over/communication can be poor.
- How does the practice arrange special services for elderly people?
- Who does the screening?
- Is screening available for those under 65?
- What do they screen for?
- Does the practice have regular liaison meetings with the Community Mental Health Team (CMHT) for the elderly?
- Will they visit the housebound on a twice-yearly basis?
- What procedures does the practice have for medication reviews and pharmacy advice?

Primary care services

Primary care is the term used to indicate those health services delivered in the local community. The GP and the services provided in the practice or health centre are key elements in primary care, but new organisations, Primary Care Trusts (PCTs), have been developed to coordinate community health services. The PCTs include a Board of Directors (including, for example, Chief Executive, Director of Nursing, Medical Director, Finance Director, etc.) and local GPs so that GPs are closely involved in monitoring, improving and expanding services. PCTs are usually responsible for district nursing, health visiting and the newly developing intermediate care services.

Intermediate care

Intermediate care is a government initiative that has broad and narrower definitions:

'An approach to health care intended to facilitate patients' transitions from home-managed chronic impairment to institution-based dependence, or to help terminally ill people be as comfortable as possible at the end of their lives.'

Also:

'That range of services designed to facilitate transition from hospital to home, and from medical dependence to functional independence, where the objectives of care are not primarily medical, the patient's discharge destination is anticipated, and a clinical outcome of recovery (or restoration of health) is desired.'

Intermediate care therefore includes convalescence, respite and rehabilitation. Schemes for older people include community hospitals, hospital at home schemes (hospital admission avoidance including acute and post-acute treatment, particularly post-surgical), rapid response teams (hospital admission avoidance with emphasis on flexibility, personal care and rehabilitation), hospital supported discharge teams, stroke rehabilitiation outreach teams and nurse-led outreach and support teams in the nursing/residential sector.

All of these exciting possibilities are in the development phase with currently little evidence for evaluation of effectiveness, cost benefit, etc. There will be local variability, but one of the hallmarks is flexibility. The General Practitioner will be one main source of information about local projects and schemes suitable for clients with issues needing resolving around their confusion, for example respite, acute or chronic illness, mobility decline, continence, etc. The other resource will be the local Primary Care Trust and/or social services department, as it is hoped that many schemes will be community based (an intermediate care centre) and joint health and social care developed.

The schemes do need careful evaluaton to ensure that there is no ageism in access and that staff are skilled in elderly care. The intention is that they provide new and needed resources, not cheaper and less effective resources than a well-equipped hospital site. They should form part of the total umbrella of care and not necessarily replace any one specific area.

Practice and district nurses

Practice nurses are based in the GP surgery and carry out a range of duties – for example, wound dressing, blood pressure monitoring, health promotion – usually via a separate booking/clinic system.

District nurses are fully qualified nurses who have undergone specialist community nurse training. Their job is a particularly hard yet rewarding one. A group of nurses usually work out of a GP practice, allowing good communication between the two groups of professionals. The work is highly varied, from treating ulcers and wounds, supervising medication, giving injections and monitoring diabetes to advising on incontinence. There are also specialist nurses (clinical nurse specialists) in wounds care, diabetes and incontinence, as well as specialist palliative care nurses. They often become involved with the most dependent and chronically ill clients and become a source of social support as well as expert advice during their contact period.

Some of the less skilled aspects of nursing have been given over to other groups, such as bathing attendants, who usually offer a weekly service – which requires its own particular skills. This service is organised by social services. Access to the nursing service is usually through the GP, although you can refer yourself directly by phoning the district nursing headquarters, listed under the Health Authority.

Whatever services visit an elderly person, they and the carer should keep a note of the person's name and a telephone number where they can be contacted. The services are usually very conscientious and aware of the responsibility that is placed upon them. However, sometimes things do go wrong (especially in times of financial constraint), and then there can be nothing worse than wondering if a service is going to appear or not. A phone call can solve the problem or at least afford communication with the agency involved.

Mental health services

All hospital and community mental health services have been reorganised under the management of Mental Health Trusts. There is local variation, but usually in-patient beds (voluntary and under Sections 2 and 3 of the Mental Health Act) are within psychiatric hospitals or specialised units in general hospitals. Community services are coordinated via recently established Community Mental Health Teams (CMHTs) for under-65s and over-65s.

Community Mental Health Teams

An interactive multidisciplinary approach is central to the philosophy that provision of comprehensive, co-ordinated and continuous community care for people with severe and long-term mental health problems should be delivered through a 'principle' vehicle with a single point of entry to varied services. This 'vehicle' has been defined as the Community Mental Health Team, which is often based in buildings separate from hospital settings, referred to as the Community Mental Health Centres (CMHCs). We have lagged somewhat behind our colleagues in the United States, who defined and set up CMHTs as early as 1963 with specific legislation. Later, 'case management' was introduced to co-ordinate a range of appropriate services.

Traditionally, old age psychiatry has practised multidisciplinary assessment, usually in the patient's home to gain maximum information about the circumstances of clients. The former consultant-led service has now been superseded by a generic assessment, still usually in the community, which is fed back to the team at weekly or twice-weekly meetings. Various models of team structure, process and integration have been advanced since the early 1990s. Structure refers to the composition of a team and how it is managed. Process describes how referrals are received and how the team works with service users over time. Integration refers to the closeness or working between members.

CMHTs require a team leader (who can come from any medical or social services background) who must oversee the collective responsibility for the team's specified objectives. These include ensuring that all cognitively impaired clients receive a medical examination and that collateral history is sought; liaising with social services, day centres, benefit offices, etc.; implementing occupational therapy assessments to assess level of capability; making sure that medical problems are dealt with by the GP or a medical specialist in elderly care; making sure that placement issues are addressed; checking capacity to consent and make wills, etc.; reviewing financial problems and taking suitable action; monitoring medication; and allocating patient counselling to community psychiatric nurses. The goal should be to integrate the various parts of what have been, up until now, fragmented services. The process most teams adopt is based on logical stages:

- publicising the service and providing optimal means of access
- deciding on appropriate referrals
- receiving referrals in a way that allows the effective planning of assessment or an emergency response when necessary
- determining criteria for acceptance for assessment
- allocating referrals for assessment
- assessment
- acceptance for longer-term work
- allocation for longer-term work
- intervention and/or monitoring
- team review and support

These team processes have provided a useful framework for service development, but as we write staffing and structures have not been agreed nationally. The budgets for teams are also still in a state of flux, with as yet no date for the merger of health and social services budgets. As of 1st April 2001 CMHTs had to be established and operating some system of single point access to elderly mental health services. Anyone can make a referral just by phoning and asking their GP to write a letter.

Some likely team structures and location of bases

In a survey conducted in the mid-1990s by the Sainsbury Centre the team bases were found to be, in order of most to least common:

- Community Mental Health Centre (purpose-built)
- in-patient unit or hospital site
- day centre or day hospital
- community resource centre
- other

An out-of-hours service is likely to be provided by CMHTs in the future. Emergency assessment on the whole is via domiciliary assessment or presentation at Accident and Emergency, where the casualty officer may refer on to a specialist in medicine or psychiatry. CMHTs offer multi-disciplinary assessment and team discussion of referred patients. Therefore the client may initially be seen by any member of the team and a generic history is taken and fed back to the team meeting, which most teams conduct on a weekly basis. The appropriate service, follow-up or reassessment is then decided upon. The needs of dementia patients are complex and therefore the assessment process can take some time, but this is in the patient's interest in the longer term. Most teams have the following members – those listed in brackets are less common:

- consultant psychiatrists
- junior doctors – usually a senior house officer in training (2–3 years post-qualification) and/or a specialist registrar who is more experienced (4–8 years post-qualification)
- a trust grade doctor, for example associate specialist
- social workers
- community psychiatric nurses
- support workers
- administrative staff

- (psychologists)
- (occupational therapists)
- (speech therapists)
- (interpreters)
- (physiotherapists)

A number of professionals such as continence advisors, dentists, hearing specialists and opticians can be accessed via the team but are not an intrinsic part of it. Most importantly, higher levels of intervention, such as day hospitals, in-patient assessment and the memory clinic can be accessed via the CMHT.

The role of the community psychiatric nurse (CPN)

These nurses are specially trained in psychiatry and usually in general nursing as well. They are known as CPNs and work full-time in the community supporting people with all types of psychiatric disorder, including dementia. They are divided into those working with the 18–65 age group and those working with the over-65s. They are highly specialised and cover the whole range of mental illness, offering help and support to sufferers of and carers of those with psychosis (late onset schizophrenia), depression, anxiety disorders and dementia. A lot of their work involves coping with crises, making first assessments for the CMHT and then monitoring the situation. This often means liaising with social services and GPs for help and advice.

Day hospitals

The primary function of a day hospital is assessment, investigation and management of medical problems (care of elderly day hospitals) or mental health problems (psychiatry of old age hospitals) when in-patient admission is not necessary. Multidisciplinary working is the norm, with access to specialties outside the core groups. Most day hospitals are only open on week days, though out of hours and weekend opening are developing. Transport to and from the unit can be arranged. Carers can be interviewed and their needs addressed.

Psychiatric day hospitals work with disordered behaviour, aggression, medication difficulties and sleep disorders, and they also give support whilst diseases like dementia, depression and psychosis are investigated. Problems with incontinence involve close liaison with the continence nurse advisor. Special groups can help with skills such as reality orientation, which involves relearning the day, the date and current affairs. Carers can be taught to help the elderly person in this process by repeatedly reminding and reassuring them of where they are. Demented patients live in the past because they can access long-term memories more easily than newer present-day ones. The therapy uses the most recent clear memory the patient has as a starting point and works forwards to the present day, reinforcing things that are particularly helpful to daily life. A psychologist can be invaluable in working with this type of client.

Increasingly day hospitals provide outreach teams to fulfil assessment and therapy functions in the client's home. The expansion of the team approach to providing help in the client's home forms the central part of a new government initiative, intermediate care.

Memory clinics

It is clear to anyone involved with elderly people that the worry of developing memory loss and dementia is great indeed. Some of this worry stems from a knowledge of how the elderly mentally confused have, in the past, been looked after by the 'system'. A picture of bewildered old people dressed in food-stained clothes and wandering aimlessly, unattended to by properly trained carers is strong, and it cannot be denied that it is somewhere close to the truth in certain places. The other reason for this worry is the general lack of knowledge about memory loss and dementia. This ignorance leads to untold fear.

The first memory clinics were established in the 1980s, but they remain a comparatively rare resource. Their role is to investigate people presenting with memory impairment and help with reversible and irreversible causes of the dementia syndrome. Although most referrals come via the GP, some self-referrals are accepted. A number of the worried will present to such clinics, but they too should be given an assessment, since this in itself can be reassuring, especially if there is a family history of dementia. GPs are increasingly conscious of memory problems, particularly in the light of headlines about treatments for dementia. Detection, however, is often delayed until the disease is more severe. Once a memory clinic is up and functioning, the number of referrals often exceeds what can be dealt with quickly, and a waiting list develops. It is a staff- and time-consuming business to run a memory clinic well, but many function very effectively, and most are very proactive. Where available they are usually the first choice of referral for a GP who suspects memory loss in a patient.

The clinic should operate not only as a place of diagnosis and possible treatment but also as a community resource, offering advice and counselling, relative support groups (often within the day hospital setting) and access to social services. The types of professionals employed will vary from clinic to clinic, and there are many different models operating. Expect to see, at the very least, a doctor and a nurse specialising in dementia. Additionally, psychometric testing (see page 94), often carried out by a psychologist, and help from the occupational therapist and a social worker are now common. Assessment is usually performed independently, with histories and investigation results pooled at a team meeting to arrive at a diagnosis and review problem areas.

Psychologists are often involved when it is not entirely clear whether memory loss is present or not, since they have batteries of specialised tests to uncover hidden problems. Different psychologists use different tests, but they are all designed to test for short-term memory loss, attention and concentration, naming, fitting things together, IQ, reaction time, etc. Some centres use computers to help with these tests, and patients often enjoy being 'examined' by them. The psychiatrist/physician will look for reversible causes of dementia, and will review the patient's mental state to exclude a diagnosis of depression. Many elderly people presenting with depression or psychosis for the first time have an underlying dementia which is revealed once the depression is treated.

Secondary care services

These are the services supplied by acute hospital trusts, general hospitals and teaching hospitals. They usually include the departments of health care of the elderly, neurology and general medicine. To all of these, people with confusion may be referred. The acute trusts run the Accident and Emergency departments and the out-patient clinics of the above specialties.

NHS Direct

This is a confidential 24-hour telephone helpline staffed by expert nurses. By calling 0845 4647 you can speak to a nurse for advice at any time of the day or night, wherever you are in the UK. You can expect your call to be answered quickly. There will be an interpreter to provide advice in your own language if you need this. There is also an Internet site, NHS Direct Online (for the address see Appendix 2, page 180).

LOCAL AUTHORITY
Social services

- social workers/welfare assistants (community and hospital based)
- care/case managers (review on-going need for help and support)
- access to residential and nursing homes (permanent and respite)
- meals on wheels
- home care (help with washing, dressing, bathing, some meal preparation)
- day centres and luncheon clubs
- day and night sitting services (e.g. Crossways)
- incontinence laundry services
- community occupational therapy

The local authority employs social workers (and unqualified care assistants) who are the key advisers concerning the range of social services available to help as well as advice on benefits.

A social worker can be a tremendous resource to a family or patient in difficulty, who will act as an advocate, representing the patient when systems seem daunting. They often work with more vulnerable, frail individuals who live alone. They can help with the basics of form filling and provide the human contact element that should also not be overlooked. Whilst someone is in hospital, it is obligatory that they have access to a social worker.

Social work falls into two main areas: practical (organising home care packages such as home helps, meals on wheels and benefit advice) and counselling (providing emotional support in bereavement issues, moving into residential care, dealing with serious illness). Most social workers possess these skills; what they do not possess is the time needed to deal with the complex problems that the elderly often have. One of the scandals of our time is the absence of sufficient supportive legislation for the elderly population and their social care needs. Any confused elderly person should have access to a social worker.

Support at home can avoid hospital admission, which can further disable and disorientate an already confused individual. The provision of a good home care (and it must be said that home care is of variable quality and reliability) is prob- ably the most important aspect of keeping a mentally confused person at home. What home care can and cannot do is increasing proscribed; however, most will clean, do a small amount of shopping and laundry, and perhaps help to prepare a meal. These tasks, together with the human contact they provide, means that thousands of people have less lonely and more fulfilling lives. Withdrawing this service, if a home help is sick or it is a public holiday, often means that someone is admitted to hospital.

Meals on wheels provide one hot meal a day. The meals are not to everyone's liking and you may have to pay for them. They are generally supplied five to seven times a week. Most areas now cater for special dietary or religious requirements such as diabetic, Kosher and Halal food.

Day centres both for the general elderly population and for elderly mentally infirm (EMI) clients are run by social services and provide some of the benefits of meals on wheels and home helps. A hot meal is provided as well as companionship. Many provide transport and arrange outings as well as specialist advice in the centre itself. They should be recreational and diversional. Some will tolerate disruptive behaviour, but they cannot usually deal with incontinence. Some will provide a bathing and personal care service. They can provide welcome respite for carers. Few are responding to the call to open at weekends, with the notable exception of Jewish Care. Some NHS day hospitals for dementia now open on Saturdays.

Sitting services are becoming more available and are popular. They allow the carer to go out for a few hours and have time to themselves, whilst someone sits in looking after the frail or confused person. This can be a one-off or a regular service. Some areas offer a night sitting service so that a carer can get an undisturbed night's sleep. The benefits are obvious, but there are a few drawbacks – although sitters do have training, if there is no rapport between client and sitter things can be fraught.

Telephones often form a lifeline between an elderly person and their carers and services. However, it is still true that not every old person has a telephone, and perhaps more importantly an alarm linked to it. With the alarm system a person wears a pendant around their neck which in times of emergency is activated and notifies a central control room. The control room tries to contact the person at home (in case the alarm has been triggered accidentally or if the person is lonely and just wants to talk), but if there is no reply two helpers are dispatched in a car to see what has happened and take action if necessary. This is an invaluable aid and gives peace of mind to both the elderly person and their relatives.

Community occupational therapists provide an assessment service where aids and adaptations to the home are needed. In cases of frailty, or confusion that requires constant supervision, they assess the person actually in their home and arrange for the adaptations to be carried out. These may be minor, such as putting blocks under the chair legs to make chairs easier to get out of, or major, such as the provision of a purpose-built bathroom or a stair lift for more disabled people.

Who pays?

Local Authorities are responsible for managing the financial budgets of home care managers and for accessing and arranging the finances associated with entering a residential or nursing home. The budget for institutional care is held by the Local Authority. Health authorities can pay for some of the nursing home costs in special circumstances.

In England and Wales services provided can be and are charged for – there is discretion over home care charges. For residential and nursing home care the client is means tested using a financial statement of financial assets. If you are assessed as having savings (currently over £11,500), then you will have to pay an increasing proportion of costs towards your care, either at home or in institutions. For institutional care your assets are assessed for the seven years *prior* to your need so that claimants cannot gain state benefits by transfering assets to relatives. Benefits, such as Disability Living Allowance (DLA) and Attendance Allowance together with state and contributory pensions are also taken into account and may be used to help pay for care that is received.

This area is extraordinarily complex and advice should always be sought. Residential care has always been means tested; however, the public disquiet concerning nursing home charges has been unabated since the Conservative government of the late 1980s altered the care environment. They gradually closed (free) NHS beds used for long-term care and rapidly expanded the private nursing home sector. Initially the government paid the nursing home bill, but when it escalated they introduced means testing, without public debate.

In Scotland, an extraordinary experiment is being implemented. In July 2000 the long-term care policy (part of the NHS plan), which arose out of a Royal Commission on this subject, was debated. The Government rejected the

Commission's central proposal that personal care in institutions should be free at the point of use for all, irrespective of means. Westminster plumped for the main recommendation of the minority report that only *nursing* care should be free. The politics following the death of Donald Dewar resulted in a revolt in Scotland and a reversal of policy, meaning that the Scottish decision will provide a controlled experiment in just how expensive it is to provide personal care free to frail elderly people. The Royal Commission estimated that the cost for personal and nursing care in Britain would be a modest £1.1 billion per annum (1995 prices) rising to £6.4 billion per annum by 2051. Most of this is for direct personal care, such as help with washing, dressing, eating and moving around, and does not include the preparation of meals. The Commission estimated that making all nursing care free would initially cost £220 million per annum.

The problem is two-fold: there is not a workable definition of the difference between nursing care and personal care and in England the current legislation is perceived to be unfair to those in institutional care who have savings or their own home. Why, people ask, should I have to sell my house and deny my children a legacy when others, who have been 'feckless', get long-term care free? At present there are very few long-term care insurance policies in existence (34,000 at the end of 1999). Insurers have difficulty promoting a product most of us would like to deny that we will ever need, and which may in any case be very bad value for money. One solution is for the Government to agree to pay for care after a fixed period, say three to four years. This would make it easier for insurers to price the risk. Clearly it is unfair to have one system in Scotland and another elsewhere, but if the past is anything to go by the future is likely to offer several more U-turns.

The government has yet to decide finally the scheme it

will use to pay for some nursing care within the residential/ nursing sectors in England. One proposal is that the care provided by registered nurses would be free, but not that provided by healthcare assistants. The nursing needs of older people are expected to have to undergo an assessment process. Following this, they may be divided into three bands. Those needing least care would get a small subsidy and those needing most care a higher subsidy. The new finalised rules are due to come into operation in October 2001.

Residential care (Part III accommodation)

A large number of residential (Part III) care homes used to be owned, staffed and managed by the Local Authority. This is increasingly rare as Local Authorities move towards commissioning and monitoring standards provided by the independent sector. The term Part III derives from Part III of the National Assistance Act 1948 that set care homes up. At the end of the 1980s they remained the main provider of care for the elderly frail. These dreaded 'old people's homes' with workhouse connotations, like the old mental hospitals, needed an overhaul.

The original concept of old people's homes was to provide the level of care that a relative could reasonably be expected to provide. This was fine until the number of older frail people began to rise over and above provision of care homes and their disabilities increased. The homes were not designed for, or staffed in sufficient numbers to cope with, the increasing number of residents who were mentally or physically infirm. Add to that the problems of mobility and mental confusion, coupled with poor staff training, and there was a recipe for disaster. Redesign, with smaller units, single and double rooms, one or two levels with lift access and secure 'wandering' areas has improved these environments for residents and made them safer and more suitable for staff to work in.

Access to residential (and nursing) care

Most local authorities use a panel system for administrating admission to institutional care. The elderly person is financially assessed and reports are submitted by health and social services putting the case for the use of an expensive resource. A social worker must be allocated and must submit their report to a panel, which collectively decides whether a home care package, sheltered housing scheme or institutional care is most appropriate.

Not infrequently, following an admission to hospital institutional care is recommended. This usually follows a multidisciplinary assessment by a hospital team headed by a consultant and a recommendation that care at home is no longer appropriate. If a patient is so confused that they continuously call out or are behaviourally disruptive to other people (given that it is their home too), they will not be accepted into ordinary residential care and will need to be placed in a home that caters for the elderly mentally infirm. It is about trying to match needs with a level of intervention that meets but does not exceed those needs. All in all a difficult, if not impossible, task given that the client's needs may fluctuate over time.

The person should visit the home before any decisions are made on either side, and many homes like a probationary visit and period of residence before they accept anyone as a permanent placement. This can be for as little as 48 hours or as long as six weeks, and gives everyone time to decide if the move is right for them.

In some residential care homes staffing levels remain dangerously low. Payment for such demanding work is derisory, making recruitment difficult and training rare. Standards are improving, but the problem of unskilled staff on poor pay makes a lot people think twice before entering into care. Recent scandals still resonate. Many people enter these institutions reluctantly, only to find life socially much better than previously and probably a lot easier. However, the decision to give up one's home is never easy, even when it is clear that the individual cannot cope. There is anguish and guilt on the part of carers. The whole process is fraught and can seem intolerable. Detailed discussion may need to take place via a case conference.

Much research has been done into residential care. Although clients may enter continent and mobile, problems do develop. Most surveys indicate that at least half of the residents are incontinent of urine and at least a quarter are severely mentally confused. Specialist homes catering for the severely confused (elderly mentally infirm – EMI) have higher staff ratios and staff are trained in dementia and behaviour disorders. Clients are allowed to wander, problem behaviours are tackled and different regimes are used to avoid or cope with incontinence. Residential homes are registered with the Local Authority.

The following checklist gives a guide to some of the questions to be asked about when institutional care is being considered:

• What are the rules and regulations?
• Can the client bring some of their own furniture?
• What are the services for guests (over-night stays)?
• What types of room or accommodation are available?
• What arrangements does the home have for medical (GP/psychiatrist) cover?
• Are there sufficient numbers of trained staff and helpers?
• Does the home have a happy atmosphere? (check the communal areas)
• Are there activities, and if so, how often?
• What would the staff do if the patient's physical or mental health worsened?
• Can the home respond to cultural/spiritual needs?
• Is the case of minority ethnic residents are there staff who can communicate with them?

Long-stay hospital bed versus nursing home provision

Following the rapid expansion of the private nursing home sector, the number of continuing care (long-stay) beds within departments of elderly care medicine rapidly declined. Most departments have some beds for the most severely physically (and usually mentally) frail elderly. What constitutes a need for a long stay (continuing care) hospital bed and what constitutes a need for nursing home care is decided locally. If an elderly person's needs are deemed to require a permanent stay in hospital, then this must be provided for. This situation has led to friction between hospital authorities and some families since residential and nursing care are means tested, whilst NHS continuing care leaves the patient's assets intact. Long-stay hospital patients are severely physically and mentally disabled and require ongoing nursing and medical care. The difference between the two types of client can sometimes be difficult for families to understand, so each area now has arbitration plans which can resolve disputes in the care pathway. Usually, with clear guidance from health and social services, differences can be easily resolved. Transparency should be looked for in these protocols.

Nursing home care

Clients who have lost mobility, i.e. who cannot walk or transfer with minimum help from a wheelchair to a bed or toilet, are usually deemed too frail for residential care. This immobility plus other care needs such as help with continence (managing incontinence), feeding, pressure area care and dressing/undressing all mean that care in a nursing home is needed. A nursing home must employ a qualified nurse to carry out and supervise nursing duties. The home must be registered with the local health authority and regularly inspected. Unfortunately, most nursing homes currently cannot manage developing illnesses – for example dehydration, chest/urine infection – and older people frequently get sent to hospital.

Promising signs in a home are the absence of unpleasant smells, sufficient staff, a pleasant atmosphere, good GP cover, the use of care plans, and daily assessments and interventions such as frequent oral fluids, bowel and urine care, pressure area inspection, monitoring of diet, etc.

Although most nursing homes are excellent, some will simply transport a client to casualty at the smallest hint of worsening illness or dependency, only then to refuse to have them back. This may mean that the elderly person is admitted to a hospital miles from where they were previously living and can cause problems for everyone concerned.

This said, if you have vetted a private care home, have visited several times, and the client has had a trial period of residency and is satisfied, then it can turn out to be a good choice. Specialist private housing is also on the increase – mainly in the form of purpose-built accommodation for the frail but not very incapacitated person. Some schemes are like sheltered housing, with a warden; others have obvious adaptations in place (bath rails, hoists, stair lifts, alarms, etc.). Other schemes envisage a retirement 'village' with amenities suited to the older person and excluding younger people. On balance, choose somewhere close to family and services that you are familiar with, and predict a change of circumstances. Help can be obtained from leaflets, books and care-givers concerned with this specific issue.

Housing services

Housing is often taken for granted until a family member becomes either mentally or physically disabled. The problems associated with stairs and lifts then become very apparent. With confused elderly people there are other areas of concern, such as the person wandering out onto a busy road or disturbing the neighbours by knocking on the door. It can be difficult to install aids and adaptions in small rooms because of carer and wheelchair access, whilst larger houses become empty shells once the family have moved out and a partner has died.

Public and private housing each have their own set of problems. If you own your own home, think well in advance about its suitability should you become disabled as you age. The layout of the house is only one part of the equation. The closeness of friends and relatives is very important, especially when an informal network is needed in a crisis. Shops, parks, leisure facilities and transport, all have to be taken into account (by that fortunate section of the population who have choice in these matters).

Although the public sector is very stretched and appropriate housing is a high premium, housing departments will do all they can to move people into more suitable accommodation – ground floor flats with a garden being top of the list, or perhaps upper-floor sheltered accommodation with a lift.

'Sheltered accommodation' means different things to different people, but essentially there should be a resident or nearby warden who acts as a 'relative' and calls in nearly every day. Each resident has his or her own flat, with an alarm providing 24-hour cover. Although the warden may not be available 24 hours a day, seven days a week, some sort of emergency cover should be available, perhaps through the local police station. This relatively low level of supervision usually does not work for the confused person in the longer term.

Although many wardens do much more than their allotted time, problems often surface (as with home care) during periods of leave or illness. Bear in mind that nothing is forever, not even new warden-controlled accommodation.

DEPARTMENT FOR WORK AND BENEFITS

The process of obtaining state benefits to which you are entitled can be lengthy and complicated. This must never stop anyone from trying – there are many people willing to help fill in the forms correctly and advise you. The books and leaflets provided by the government can be helpful, but most people need extra explanation.

We suggest that if it all looks too much you ask someone from one of the voluntary agencies or your social worker to give you a hand. If you fail first time, enlist the help of your local doctor or anyone at the hospital involved in your care. There are benefits that should not be missed if you are eligible:

- Attendance Allowance
- Invalid Care Allowance
- Disability Living Allowance (DLA) (mobility and care components)
- War Disablement Pension
- Income Support

Attendance Allowance

Attendance allowance is a weekly cash sum paid to the disabled person themselves if they need help or supervision because of either physical or mental disability. The money can be spent on anything or anyone. Awards are based on the care you need, not the care you are actually getting. If you claim Attendance Allowance you have to show that you have met the conditions for needing attention and/or supervision for six months before the benefit can be awarded to you. A terminally ill claimant (who is suffering from a progressive disease and can reasonably be expected to die within six months as a result of that disease) is deemed to satisfy the conditions for the higher rate of attendance allowance and to have done so for the last six months. Advanced Alzheimer's disease (and related conditions) fall into the category of terminal diseases. There are special rules if a recipient is admitted to hospital or if they receive regular respite care – please check regularly with the benefits adviser.

Invalid Care Allowance

Invalid Care Allowance is a weekly sum paid to carers if they are spending at least 35 hours a week looking after or supervising someone who also receives the higher or middle rate of the *care* component of DLA, Attendance Allowance or Constant Attendance Allowance, in respect of industrial or war disablement. The carer must not be gainfully employed or in full-time education, and cannot be under 16 or over 65 years old.

Disability Living Allowance (DLA) (mobility and care components)

These benefits to severely disabled people were reorganised in April 1992. DLA is divided into two parts, payable at different rates, the higher rate dependent upon the claimant receiving the care component first. The old Mobility Allowance and Attendance Allowance for those under 65 have been incorporated into this new benefit.

Claimants complete extensive self-assessment claim forms (we would not advise you to do this without guidance), and most claims are then decided without medical examination. Decision-making is by an adjudication officer, who may review the case from time to time by a visit to the patient's home. Doctors review the submissions centrally. There is the right to review by tribunal if successive submissions fail.

The upper age limit for the mobility and care components

of DLA is 65, thereafter the Attendance Allowance kicks in. However, the DLA, once awarded, is for a specified duration and no longer for life, except in exceptional circumstances. If you are turned down and you are a rightful claimant you should appeal.

War Disablement Pension may be awarded to people who have been injured or disabled as result of service in Her Majesty's armed forces. Comprehensive help is available via the Pensioner's Guide (to ask for a copy phone 08456 065 065 or visit their web site www.info4pensioners.gov.uk).

Income Support

If you qualify, Income Support tops up your income to a prescribed level. If you can make a successful claim for Income Support you qualfy for the Minimum Income Guarantee (MIG). (See Appendix 2)

Voluntary organisations

The voluntary sector has well organised local schemes often with a national profile and can be helpful with support groups and befriending as well as offering advice on accessing services. They have been at the coalface and know the ropes! Try looking up the following in the phone book:

- Alzheimer's Society
- Help the Aged
- Age Concern
- Citizen's Advice Bureau
- Jewish Care

Voluntary organisations can be invaluable sources of expertise, especially in complex situations such as providing appropriate and sensitive help to older ethnic minority clients. Information and literature is often available in locally appropriate languages.

6

Assessing and Investigating Memory Loss

This chapter will address the process that a person referred for a memory problem will undergo in order to establish as accurate a diagnosis as possible. As previously indicated, dementia is a complex disorder requiring a great deal of thought and co-ordination of services to help the sufferer and their carers. There will be variations in practise from area to area, but the essentials are laid out here in order to help navigate what at times will seem a daunting and unending process.

Dementia can be assessed in both a hospital/clinic (memory clinic) and a home (domicilary) setting. Bear in mind that the needs of the patient and care-giver cannot always be fully appreciated in a clinic environment. Behavioural disturbances, such as delusions and agitation, may worsen when the patient leaves the familiarity of home. Patients may also be initially unwilling to go to a clinic. In such cases a community assessment can clarify unresolved issues and uncover specific needs.

Around 70 diseases can cause dementia. As mentioned before, three conditions are responsible for 80 per cent of cases: Alzheimer's disease, vascular dementia and dementia associated with Lewy bodies. Whether performed at home or in a clinic, evaluation of dementia requires careful observation of the patient over time. Assessment begins the moment the assessor meets the patient for the first time and then during casual conversation. Information about walking, posture, language skills, use of the hands and mood contributes to the overall understanding and helps with the diagnosis. For example, a patient may have difficulty deciding where to sit, there may be pauses when they cannot find the correct words, their walking may be slowed or they may have an odd posture, indicating that the disease has progressed to a point where motor functions (movements) are affected. Formal testing of memory and cognition can indicate areas of poor functioning and an occupational therapist's Activities of Daily Living assessment will back up any initial findings. The history from a carer or close relative is essential, since some patients cannot give an accurate account of their difficulties or may be in denial of problems because they are fearful.

The assessment of dementia in the community setting

A home visit should be carefully planned with the carer and/or patient so that maximum benefit is gained and as little stress as possible generated. This will be the first stage of building up a relationship (therapeutic alliance) so – if acceptable – as many members of the family as possible should be involved. Some information will be collected before the visit so that the assessor can concentrate on collecting accurate data. A first assessment can last anything up to an hour and a half, but a skilled interviewer may be 'in and out', so don't put too much store in the amount of time spent with the patient initially, since this is only the beginning of a process, not a one-off. Most community mental health teams will have a generic (all purpose) assessment form to make sure that the general points are covered. The whole purpose of a home visit is to take account of the total environment in which the patient functions. It is not just a medical review but a social one too – a holistic approach. The assessment is fed back to the whole team who then comment upon specific or general points and devise an action plan.

The following is a brief outline of the assessment used by mental health teams for elderly people. It covers a broad spectrum of topics:

- referral letter
- general information about the patient
- agencies involved
- reason for referral – client's account/informant's account/ expectations
- family history
- personal history
- personality before they were ill
- past mental health history
- past medical history
- current medical history
- current physical state/any physical abnormalities
- medication/allergies
- description of accommodation – condition/security/ dangers/ signs of incontinence or abuse
- financial situation – pension/allowances/worries
- services currently provided
- mental state examination – appearance/behaviour/speech/ mood/sleep/odd thoughts and hallucinations/memory and concentration/suicidal ideas/insight.
- nursing assessment/level of dependence – walking/dressing/continence/feeding/cooking/shopping/managing finances
- support network

- risk assessment – care programme approach (low or high risk)
- comments on matters not yet covered – patient and carer
- services needed but not available
- the mini mental state examination
- initial action plan
- referral to other services (immediate)

Clearly not everything can be done on an initial assessment, but it acts as a starting point for the rest of the process. What follows is best performed, or can only be performed, by a visit to a specialist clinic, although the GP may be able to organise routine blood tests from their surgery. Some of the work must be done at a hospital since this is where the technology is located.

The assessor will almost certainly ask for a medical review if the diagnosis is not clear from the initial impression. The doctor will be keen to know about the history of the illness over the last few years or months. It is helpful when going to the clinic to cast your mind back to the length of time symptoms have been present and try to be honest with yourself about this. Things like a sudden onset or rapid progression are extremely important to know about since they may point to significant diagnoses.

Talking to doctors

Some patients and carers find talking to a doctor a difficult experience: they often feel that they have not expressed themselves well or conveyed their true feelings or anxieties to the clinician. Doctors are now being trained to see communication as a vital skill so that even where a doctor is not a naturally good communicator and the patient nervous, progress can be made. GPs are the gatekeepers to so many services and forms of help that good and effective communication with them is essential. Hopefully most GPs have a good working relationship with their patients. In a few cases this does not happen; the fault may be on either side, but a patient or carer can be disadvantaged or blocked by an insensitive GP. The only way forward is adequate dialogue, putting the issue as openly as possible. If a service is refused, ask the GP to explain why such a service or treatment is not available at this point in time. If you are still not satisfied with the answers you are getting, most practices now have an internal complaints procedure and offer another GP for a discussion of the issues. It may be that transfer to another practice is necessary, but that is obviously not a guarantee that the matter will be resolved to your satisfaction. Once a referral has been sent to a secondary care facility such as a Community Mental Health Team, day hospital or memory clinic, a service may not be co-ordinated by a doctor but rather a service manager, who will discuss urgency with a senior medical practitioner. If the GP deems the case urgent, referrals can be seen within 48 hours for home assessment.

It used to be the case that only a GP could refer for an expert opinion. However, the culture in the NHS is altering in favour of self-referral, particularly in mental health, with the CMHTs as single points of access. Private referrals (where a fee is paid) can still be made directly to an individual consultant or private hospital in many areas. We would advise getting the GP to write to your local service initially. If there is a problem with either the GP or access, it may be possible in some areas to self-refer, but only 50 per cent of CMHTs accepted such referrals at the survey in the mid-1990s. Most GPs, however, are not unreasonable about organising a specialist opinion. One is always a patient of a GP first and foremost; a specialist will advise on diagnosis and management once a patient is under the combined care of both GP and consultant.

The consultant (or the image of one) can be intimidating, but remember that such individuals in psychiatry and old age medicine are generally humane sorts with a lot of time for older people – that is why they are doing this now very competitive and fashionable job!

The medical history

Once the GP has been seen, a referral sent, a home visit carried out by a community psychiatric nurse (CPN) and an initial history taken, the next step is a visit to a clinic. This is where the patient's history will be fleshed out and detailed assessment made in specific areas.

Conditions that have occurred in the past may have something to do with the present state of the patient. It is important that the doctor is told about the following:

- Any head injury – sufficient to cause the patient to be unconscious can be relevant to both Alzheimer's and normal pressure hydrocephalus. It can also cause a blood clot on the surface of the brain (subdural haematoma), which in turn causes fluctuating levels of consciousness (patients are variously alert and unresponsive).
- Epilepsy can lead to brain damage from seizures where the brain is deprived of oxygen. Some of the drugs taken for this condition can also affect intellect.
- Hypothyroidism (an under-active thyroid gland) can be significant, especially if an overactive thyroid earlier in life was treated surgically.
- Any metabolic disorder or failure of an organ should be mentioned – diabetes, heart attacks, odd heartbeat, stroke, kidney or liver disease, rheumatoid arthritis, lupus (an immune disorder) and blood disorders.
- Any past history of carcinoma (cancer), even many years before, can be relevant – especially of the lungs or breast.

- Tell the doctor about medications you are taking (with the doses).
- Past psychiatric history is very relevant (for example, depression). Current symptoms are also important.
- Be realistic about the amount of alcohol you drink and over what period.
- Your family may have a history of dementia, although familial Alzheimer's is rare. Remember anyone with Huntingdon's disease or Down's syndrome.
- The doctor will ask about your social circumstances again, since there may be things like driving and managing money that have been overlooked.

One of the questions the doctor will be asking themselves is whether the illness they are assessing is acute or chronic (see Chapters 2 and 3). The difference between delirium and dementia is an important one.

Physical examination

Clinical examination is very important, as the patient may have problems in expressing symptoms verbally. Observation of general appearance is the first rule in psychiatric practice. The doctor will do a general examination of each of the major body systems in turn, before moving on to the mental state examination previously described and the mini mental state examination.

Investigations

Good clinical judgement is the cornerstone upon which to determine which specialist tests are required to clarify the situation. By this stage the doctor and the memory clinic team will begin to exclude treatable and reversible causes of dementia. However, not all of the causes can be excluded with a history and physical examination alone, and routine laboratory tests are necessary for most patients.

A simple haematological screen and biochemical profile can lead to surprising findings, which are often treatable. These tests are simple and every patient should have them as baseline investigations.

The following are also available in most centres:

- The Electrocardiogram (ECG) is a tracing of the rhythm of the heart and can detect abnormal rhythms and heart disease (such as previous heart attack and enlargement). It is important to know about these because abnormal heart function increases the likelihood of stroke and may indicate a need to add or delete medication.
- Chest radiograph (chest X-ray) can occasionally show evidence of unsuspected disease. Other X-rays have been superseded by CT and MRI (see opposite and page 119).
- Doppler ultrasonography is used to detect narrowing of the arteries in the neck that supply the brain. Narrowing of vessels slows and reduces blood flow, and is a good predictor of vascular dementia, but blood flow to the brain is also affected in Alzheimer's disease.
- Electroencephalography (EEG) detects the electrical activity of the brain by electrodes attached to the scalp. It is particularly useful in detecting metabolic disorders and delirium. If the whole brain is diseased (as in Alzheimer's) typical changes are seen on the recording. Very particular changes are also seen with new variant CJD, the human form of bovine spongiform encephalopathy (BSE). This investigation is making a comeback in some centres, since its diagnostic accuracy is very high.
- Lumbar puncture examines the fluid that surrounds the brain. It is used where infection and immune system diseases are suspected.

- Electromyography (EMG) is a way of tracing the activity of the body's large muscles, which can malfunction in some cases of brain disease. It can be useful if rare diseases are suspected, such as motor neurone disease, some metabolic diseases and multiple sclerosis.
- Syphilis is making a comeback after years of being under control. A simple blood antibody test is recommended for all patients. It is in the late stages of syphilis that the brain is affected.
- Currently HIV testing of older people is comparatively rare, although it is likely that this will increase in the future.
- Urine testing is easy and can give a lot of information. Infections are a frequent cause of acute memory difficulties and confusion in elderly people.

This battery of tests might seem excessive, but they can all be accomplished in one day if things are well organised. Not everyone will need all of these tests, but everyone should have routine blood tests, a urine test and an ECG. Most people will then require some form of brain scan (see below). The history and physical examination will give most of the information, whilst the lab tests will identify reversible causes and create a framework in which doctors can monitor the patient and perhaps predict the stage of the disease.

Brain scans (neuroimaging)

Computerised tomography (CT)
The computer uses X-rays to build up pictures of the brain. The patient lies still on a horizontal surface which moves through the machine.

The images appear as flat black and white pictures which can visualise the brain down to 2mm segments. This investigation is used to rule out tumours, vascular and accidental

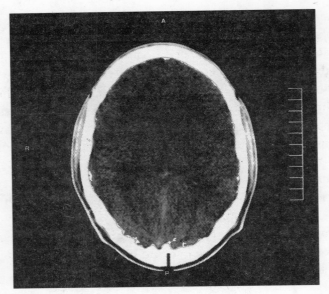

Illustration of a normal CT scan

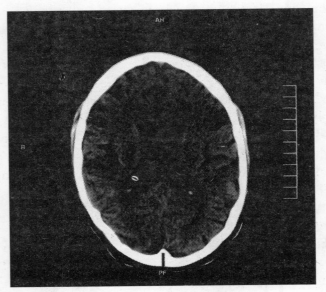

Illustration of a CT scan showing 'shrinkage' of brain
Courtesy of Dr Otto Chan, Royal London Hospital, Barts and the London Trust

damage to the brain, for example from road traffic head injuries.

Generally in Alzheimer's disease nothing remarkable is shown. However, experienced radiologists may be able to observe shrinkage of a particular part of the brain, the hippocampus. This condition indicates Alzheimer's disease as opposed to normal ageing changes and is also called medial temporal lobe atrophy (MTLA). Researchers are interested in this change, since it often comes before any noticeable memory loss occurs.

A problem of CT scanning is one of resolution (as in a blurred photograph, it is impossible to see accurately very tiny abnormalities). On balance this is still the cheapest and most widely used brain imaging technique at the beginning of the 21st century.

Magnetic resonance imaging (MRI)

This investigation is more frightening for disorientated patients because of the noise the machine makes in performing the scan. The noise is due to huge magnets being rotated rapidly at 90 degrees to each other to produce a fluctuating magnetic field. As a result the brain gives out radiation, which a computer analyses to build up a remarkably accurate picture of the living brain. This investigation is done when CT has drawn a blank but vascular disease is still suspected. Claustrophobia is currently a possible problem but a new generation of faster unenclosed scanners is being developed.

Single photon emission computed tomography (SPECT)

This investigation uses a chemical 'tag' which emits radiation to measure blood flow in different areas of the brain. This is called regional cerebral blood flow. As tracers or tags become more specific, so greater clarity of diagnosis will be possible. At present it is fronto-temporal and Alzheimer's

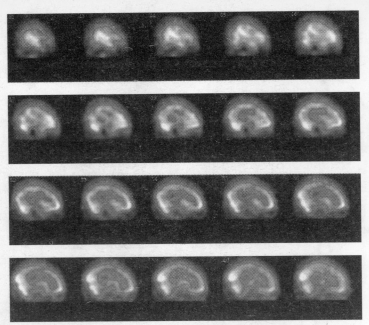

Normal SPECT scan showing uniform distribution of tracer

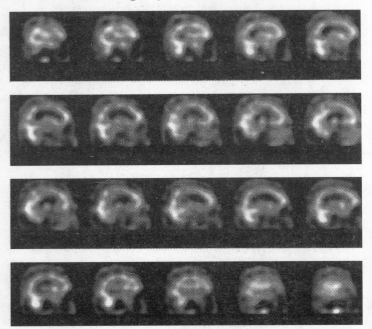

Abnormal SPECT scan showing abnormal/non-uniform distribution of tracer
Courtesy of Dr Neil Garvie, Royal London Hospital, Barts and the London Trust

disease which are being studied and mapped by this method.

Positron emission tomography (PET)

This is a very specific and expensive investigation, used only in research centres at present, which measures the metabolism in certain parts of the brain in real life and time. It can measure oxygen and regional blood flow and even look at the number of receptors in certain brain areas.

How scans help the diagnosis in dementia

Previously, CT and MRI scanning were used to exclude the possibility of tumours and strokes, and to indicate the presence of hydrocephalus. However, there is now indisputable evidence that there is significant damage to the temporal lobe of the brain in even the earliest cases of Alzheimer's disease. Whether or not a scan is performed may depend on how the disease presents – some cases are obvious. Nevertheless, some clinicians like to perform all the investigations for completeness. The tests may show nothing abnormal. This does not mean that the diagnosis is wrong – particularly if the radiologist has not looked for the tell-tale signs of medial temporal lobe shrinkage – just that it is less likely.

Clearly, in major teaching centres there will be a number of research projects going on which involve some of these very specialised scans. Where brain imaging is thought necessary, most psychiatrists rely on the CT scan for their baseline investigation.

The role of the psychologist in assessment

In the UK psychology is still a growing speciality, and not all areas of the country have a psychologist specialising in elderly care. Those that do are lucky indeed. The psychologist's role is not just to measure dementia or memory loss, but this is one of the many skills they have to offer, and some specialise in this sort of testing. They will:

- see how damaged the memory is
- find out exactly where the problem areas in thinking are
- try to suggest aids to memory and ways to manage family problems
- give a separate objective opinion so that any changes can be seen when the patient is tested in the future.

It is important for the psychologist to foster an atmosphere where the patient will do their very best and not underperform in the assessment. Psychologists are versed in setting the scene for psychological testing from the moment the patient enters the waiting area. The tests are described and the patient given feedback throughout the tasks. The assessment can take anything from 45 minutes to two hours, which may be divided into two sessions to help with fatigue.

The role of the occupational therapist in assessment

There may be significant problems around the house or in daily living tasks that still haven't been picked up. The occupational therapist is skilled in disability assessment and is able to distinguish between the patient's ability to perform basic activities of daily living, such as eating and dressing, and to perform the more complicated activities that allow for greater independence, such as managing finances. Occupational therapists help the team to understand patiently the patient's limitations.

7

Therapies and Treatments for Dementia

It is now accepted that we have entered a new era in the understanding, management and treatment of dementia, all advanced by the new drug treatments for this debilitating disease. Until the 1990s only depression, which is seen early in the disease, and behaviour problems, seen late in the disease, were amenable to drug treatment. But now the situation is different. This chapter will address those issues commonly raised by families regarding what can be done to make life more bearable for the patient and the carers.

Treatment of depression in patients with cognitive impairment and dementia

There has been a long running debate about which comes first in dementia – is it memory loss or depression? It is clear that some patients who present with depression go on to become demented. Others remain psychologically mood stable in the light of a developing memory impairment, then later become depressed. All doctors should treat depression once it is diagnosed, even if memory loss is present. The question is, does treating depression have any effect on the underlying disease of dementia? Certainly the older drugs used in cases of depression (Amitripyline and Imipramine) could lead to a worsening of memory problems because they had side effects which affect memory adversely (anticholinergic effects).

Patients who have a depressive syndrome can appear like an Alzheimer's type patient – withdrawn and retarded. But treatment lifts their mood and makes them well with no residual memory problems. Treatments which are 'activating', such as the selective serotonin reuptake inhibitors (SSRIs) or selective noradrenaline reuptake inhibitors (SNRIs), are better than the more sedating tricyclic drugs (developed in the 1950s). Most readers will have heard of Prozac, but there are now many other drugs, all equally good at treating depression in elderly patients, and they are well tolerated.

Treatment of delusions and hallucinations

These symptoms are common in Alzheimer's disease, occurring earlier rather than later. They may be the reason the patient is referred to the doctor in the fist place. Hallucinations also arise in the context of acute medical illnesses but, aside from Alzheimer's, are most commonly seen in vascular or Cortical Lewy Body disease.

Drugs called anti-psychotics (neuroleptic) medication are the main treatment once an attempt has been made to alter the patient's environment, for example by keeping their room well lit to avoid shadows and keeping noise to a minimum. With drugs there is always a trade off between potency and side effects. The anti-psychotics most favoured at the time of writing are known as 'atypical' – in the sense that they cause fewer side effects than traditional neuroleptics, which include Haloperidol.

On the whole it is better to make delusions more manageable than to try to cure them. Treatment rarely removes such thoughts from a person's mind, instead they make the person tolerate them better. In some patients side effects such as sedation are desirable, whilst in others, especially those with Cortical Lewy Body disease, neuroleptics can cause serious side effects and should be avoided. If behaviour is intolerable the questions to ask are:

- What might be causing this problem and is it more than simply a dementia?
- Can it be treated by interventions other than drugs?
- Has all medical illness been ruled out?
- Is the environment suitable, or making things worse?
- What can treatment achieve?
- If we use drugs, are we using the lowest possible dose?
- Has the patient been made worse by treatment?
- When does the team need to reassess the patient?

It must be noted that, although it may be distressing to resort to drugs, judicious use of low dose medications is the best policy. Such conditions do not last throughout the course of dementia. Most medications should be discontinued after a trial of three to six months. If the problem re-emerges then the drugs can be re-started for a further three to six months.

Acute and chronic agitation

This is a topic which exercises doctors and carers alike. These states almost always lead to referral since they are so upsetting. If a patient suddenly worsens then suspect acute infection or something like a stroke. Elaborate searches are not necessary, simple physical examination and some blood and urine tests show up most of the possible causes. The doctor should be able to diagnose precisely the type of behaviour shown and give advice about early strategy, for example has there been a recent change in environment? If so, reverse this if possible. It is sad to report that there is little scientific evidence on which to base such recommendations. On the whole, if drugs are prescribed, then a low dose of a neuroleptic plus a benzodiazepine (Diazepam or Lorazepam) are the medicines of choice. Do ask if the drugs given are sedative or can cause unsteadiness or falls. It must be added that benzodiazepines and neuroleptics can also cause disinhibition, which is clearly undesirable.

Chronic aggressive behaviour occurs in many dementias, but particularly in late-stage Alzheimer's disease and frontal dementia, where the front of the brain is primarily affected. The way in which the disease progresses means that behaviours come and go, and most problems last only a few months even when left untreated. The variation in what is reported as aggressive behaviour is remarkable in that what is tolerated by one set of carers is not by another. The following often cause families to seek help:

• wandering
• faecal incontinence (see Appendix 1, page 171)
• physical violence

Physical aggression by an Alzheimer's sufferer puts them at risk of being physically abused themselves (see page 145). Always seek help and advice if a carer is finding it difficult to control their own response to challenging behaviour by the person in their care. Pain and problems such as constipation can cause someone who cannot communicate adequately to make their needs known in other ways, for example by making noises and shouting. The doctor who is reviewing the patient will have a checklist of possible problems, which should include fractures and ulcers (internal and external). Haloperidol and chlorpromazine may be used for their sedating effects. Trazodone, once a neglected antidepressant, has made a comeback because it promotes sleep and can be used as an antidepressant for restless patients. Prozac and other SSRIs have been used for agitation. Although they are not licensed for this particular problem, it is worth the doctor considering them in some circumstances. Do not be surprised that a doctor has given someone an 'alerting' antidepressant when they are already agitated!

Benzodiazepines (for example, diazepam) have a varying press amongst doctors who treat a lot of dementia suffers. They can cause too much drowsiness and therefore increase confusion, but their use is indicated where a patient just won't sleep and is exhausted, and in cases of severe agitation. Rarely, a patient can lose all control mechanisms and become even more agitated. We have reviewed a large number of papers to try and find a consensus on the use of these drugs, but there is none. However, the following is a list of drugs that have been tried and found variously successful in reducing agitation:

- Carbemazepine
- Lithium
- Sodium valproate
- Pindolol
- Bupsirone

Symptomatic treatment of cognitive decline (Alzheimer's disease)

Textbooks are now awash with reports of the triumphs of the anticholinesterases, a group of drugs licensed for symptom relief in Alzheimer's disease and related conditions. We should not forget the resistance initially put forward against their use. Health Authorities were, and still are, unconvinced of their health and financial impact. Both areas of concern have now been vindicated by the decision of the National Institute for Clinical Excellence (NICE) to recommend that these drugs are generally available to NHS patients, with the appropriate support services (such as memory clinics).

A risk is that the explanation given of the drug's effects is too simple or too technical. It is suggested that if you require further information over and above what is provided by your GP you visit the websites of the drug companies concerned and also the National Institute for Clinical Excellence web-site at www.nice.org.uk (see Appendix 2).

The chemical journey to this point in the development of Alzheimer's medication is remarkable. It has been shown that acetylcholine the neurotransmitter (chemical messenger) in the brain is significantly reduced in Alzheimer's disease and in other dementias. The brain has another chemical, an enzyme called acetylcholinesterase (AChE), whose job it is to break down acetylcholine and stop the chemical signal transmission once it has passed from one cell to another. The three drugs which are licensed for use in the UK – Donepezil (Aricept), Rivastigmine (Exelon) and Galantamine (Reminyl) – deactivate AchE and so increase the amount of acetylcholine in the brain available for sending messages. This is useful because as Alzheimer's disease progresses, less and less acetylcholine is produced, but if an AChE inhibitor is used the acetylcholine that is produced is preserved for longer. The symptoms of the disease are alleviated to a variable degree. Patients who are diagnosed early tend to be stabilised more easily and improve from baseline. As the disease progresses and the amount of acetylcholine available for neurotransmission messages falls to below pre-treatment levels, the performance of the drug will start to decline. When the disease is severe, these drugs are unlikely to have any discernible effect.

The choice of one drug over another is a question of

individual clinical judgement and experience. There is now anecdotal evidence that if a patient begins to fail on one acetylcholinesterase inhibitor then swapping to another drug in this group may be of benefit. How long patients should remain on this medication has been indicated in the NICE guidelines, but again most clinicians will vary their practise according to individual patients. What has become clear is that strict adherence to the scores achieved on assessment scales are often not predictive of functional ability and therefore it is a global impression of the patient and their environment that is most important when assessing suitability for an anticholinesterase. However, people who score more than 12 on the mini mental state examination should be considered for a trial of medication. Decisions not to treat should be accompanied by detailed explanation. In other words, only advanced irreversible dementia should be excluded.

Non-drug treatments

The acetylcholinesterase inhibitors are a significant breakthrough, and in Chapter 8 you can read of what is in the pipeline for further drug development, but drugs are not the only treatments. There are a host of complementary treatments which should not be ignored – they can do no harm and may be beneficial, especially the herbal remedy ginkgo biloba. Aromatherapy and massage also have a place and can be extremely calming. We should not just be preoccupied with treatment in the sense of cure and recovery; there may be other different goals that improve a person's quality of life and reduce distress. The method employed is simple:

- careful assessments
- adjustment of what can realistically be adjusted
- benefit to the maximum number of stakeholders (including carers)

Assessing behaviour

Assessments must review the patient's current strengths and weakness using the psychological tests that may have helped in diagnosis. The impairments will point the way to areas that should be capitalised upon. A person's coping style (and their defence mechanisms) should indicate how they are likely to react to new circumstances. Their life story gives a context for the current situation, showing preferences and choices over a lifetime and pointing to possible future developments. The assessment must also review the carer and social network, since conflict and guilt are common and should be resolved. It may be that the main carer is also frail or the family are in financial difficulties. Behaviours which cause distress should be listed in a diary which is handed to the medical team for review.

Dealing with distressing behaviour may not mean altering the behaviour at all. If the behaviour is bizarre to some onlookers but not causing distress to carers or the client, it cannot be considered a legitimate target for therapy. Similarly, delusions or hallucinations that are mild and liveable with should not be treated, since for the most part they will recede with time. The general term 'agitation' is less useful than a precise description of the behaviour, since it will clarify the target problem precisely, for example repetitive questioning. Screaming at bath time may be viewed as 'resistance' or 'stubbornness', but maybe it is sheer panic. Is this due to a long-standing fear of drowning or exposing the body? It is unusual to stop difficult behaviour completely; it is more reasonable to reduce behaviours to tolerable levels. Many difficult behaviours are a question of perception by care-givers, and strain can be reduced by simply talking through the carer's anxieties. Experience shows that sharing personal experiences in support groups, such as those run by the Alzheimer's Society (formerly called the Alzheimer's Disease Society – details in

Appendix 2, page 180), can result in solidarity with other carers, and a lessening of personal tension.

Insight

The term 'insight' describes how much a sufferer knows or realises about their condition. Opinion is divided as to how much a person should be told about their disease. There is probably an optimal amount of information-giving somewhere in between protecting the patient (and full carer) and explaining fully what is going on. This is similar to how we now deal with cancer patients and their families. Judgement is necessary. For many, personal autonomy and disdain for a patronising attitude demands full explanation. Others are grateful for a less direct approach. Different styles are usually needed at different stages and in different situations. Denial on the part of a sufferer or carer can be helpful or crippling. Grief or self-blame for what has been lost has a myriad of courses and is rarely resolved early on. What the doctor and memory clinic team can do is instil hope and gently question to find out how much the sufferer and their family already know and what their fears are. The sufferer must be listened to at all stages of the condition, no matter how difficult it might be to understand what they are asking.

Psychological therapies

There is a growing interest in psychodynamic treatments of people with dementia at all stages, utilising those memory traces which are still accessible. However, their value is uncertain beyond subjective and anecdotal stories. There are four psychological strategies which are very helpful:

- reducing cognitive load
- training and using cues

- operant conditioning
- problem prevention

Given that we continuously have to update our memory about where we are and what we are doing, the load on our brains of what we have to know in order to function at a high level is considerable. It is useful in dementia to reduce the amount of material that the person has to know, given that the brain has only a limited capacity to learn new material in these conditions. This means that one should avoid divided attention, use short simple sentences and substitute pictures and objects for the spoken word to provide a context for conversation when interacting with dementia sufferers. This simple idea is seen in action when toilets have a picture of a toilet on them or a white board is put up where the patient will come across it frequently. Cues and prompts must be obvious and used repeatedly.

The two stages of learning which are most damaged in Alzheimer's disease are acquisition (input) and retrieval (output) of information. Information which needs to be learnt must be repeatedly reinforced. The act of recalling trace information allows it to be stored in memory banks. An example would be: 'This beeper sound means you have to go to the toilet . . . What is this beeper reminding you to do?'

Operant conditioning reinforces behaviours that are good by giving the person a reward for not doing an unwanted behaviour. An example would be a man who sexually importunes a female. He is given time with a female member of staff only if he does not importune the female patient. This is reinforced by telling him he is acting like a gentleman.

Problem prevention interrupts a sequence of actions that leads up to unwanted or distressing behaviour. Sometimes this strategy demands that you be ingenious, for example by disguising doors as windows, covering up taps, or using special locks on doors to prevent wandering.

8

Legal Aspects

Protection from abuse by carers is legally enshrined for children, but there is no such specific protection for vulnerable elderly people. The exhausted carer who makes a plea for help before they abuse their elderly demented relative will find that no help is automatically forthcoming. It has long been recognised that a minimum legal framework imposing compulsory duties on statutory bodies and perhaps individuals is long overdue. The Law Commission has recognised this and incorporated similar requirements into many of its reports on the mentally incapacitated and other vulnerable adults.

The majority of the elderly mentally frail live in the community (only about six per cent live in institutions); most of them, given the right amount of help, would like to remain there. Their carers by and large agree. Surely the approach of a caring society should be to keep as many people out of institutions as possible, and those that need either medical or social homes should then have a right of entry for their own safety and well-being. Any legislation, however, must not be seen as a way to reduce individual liberty. Admission to a home should be a positive choice for the elderly person, and if the issue is one of violence to the elderly person, then other solutions should be explored, such as the perpetrator moving out – not automatically the elderly victim.

Elderly people with dementia form the largest group whose needs require legislative safeguards. As dementia progresses they become increasingly vulnerable and their needs in terms of housing, social and health services become more pressing. Currently there is no legislation that can effectively enhance the life of a sufferer. No one can insist that the local social services provide sufficient care to allow the affected person to remain at home in comparative safety. No one can insist that a carer receives a break from caring at least once every few months. No one can insist that the housing needs of a sufferer are met to enable them to function at home with help and, hence, stay in the community. (Some people, however, think that the 1986 Disabled Persons Act *does* include some of these rights but that the Act is not being fully implemented.) The elderly mentally frail should have the same right to levels of care as other members of society. The NHS and Community Care Act 1990 legislates that assessment of an elderly person's needs must be performed if requested (by social services). Whether or not this constitutes a legal right of the person to have all the assessed needs provided for by a Local Authority remains to be seen.

There are currently numerous articles of legislation that skirt around the real problem. Nevertheless, it is extremely important to understand these, for they may be the only means to insist that practical help is provided – or they may be used against the sufferer or carer's wishes.

- Mental Health Act 1983 (being revised 2001)
- guardianship.
- Section 47 of the National Assistance Act 1948
- court of protection (public trust office)
- power of attorney
- agency
- Disabled Persons Act 1986
- the living will
- Do Not Resuscitate (DNR) orders
- abuse of elderly people
- driving
- Council Tax
- Human Rights Act (European Union)

The Mental Health Act 1983

The Mental Health Act (MHA) allows for the compulsory admission to hospital of people who, because of their mental illness, are either a danger to themselves or others, or who will get much worse unless treated. Sufferers from dementia rarely fall into these categories, though occasionally severe depression or paranoia may need compulsory admission so that the patient can recover.

If the admission of an elderly mentally ill person is to occur using the MHA, there is a prescribed format for each Section of the Act used to detain a person against their will. The request can come from the nearest relative, but is usually from a social worker specialising in the field or a GP. Two doctors have to recommend the admission, usually the patient's GP and a psychiatrist, who must be approved under Section 12(2) of the MHA 1983. This indicates that the doctor has special experience of mental illness and its treatment. Ideally the GP and the psychiatrist should have known or have prior knowledge of the patient under examination. Ultimately it is the responsibility of a social worker who has undergone special training to make the application for detention to the hospital. The social worker must consult the patient's nearest relative in all cases. Often the GP has been alerted to a serious problem by a family member and consults the social worker. They assess the situation and in turn alert the psychiatrist, who must examine the person. The whole procedure can be organised and carried out within a few hours.

Under the MHA 1983 two 'orders' are commonly used. Section 2 detains a patient for 28 days for assessment but does not prevent a patient from being treated against their will if it is in their best interests. Section 3, also known as a treatment order, detains a patient for six months and they are required by law to accept the treatment of the responsible medical officer. A patient has the legal right of appeal against their detention. Their case is heard by the Mental Health Act tribunal.

The MHA is currently under review following a Royal Commission and Department of Health directive (1999). There are two areas of special importance that are being addressed by government proposals: capacity (presence or absence of the ability to make informed decisions, especially concerning the familiar coupling that treatment is necessary for the 'health and safety of the patient' or 'the protection of others') and consent (a description that is understood by two people and may involve a procedure). This complex area is still under debate.

Guardianship

A guardianship order is issued by the Local Health Authority and is effectively a social services order. To receive guardianship the person must have a mental disorder, as defined under the Mental Health Act 1983. This must be longstanding and mean that the person needs help and guidance to manage in the community.

The application for the order is very similar to that for a compulsory admission under the Mental Health Act, i.e. usually by a close relative or social worker on the recommendation of two doctors. The guardian has to be accepted by social services – the guardian may indeed be the Local Authority – and they have the power to make the person live at a specified address, attend for medical treatment (though they cannot make them accept it) and make sure that the other agencies have access to that person. A guardianship order lasts for six months, but can be renewed. A guardian has no access to the person's money or household goods.

The Guardianship Order (sections 7–10) of the Mental

Health Act 1983 is infrequently used, possibly due to the fact that most often it is Local Authorities themselves who become the guardians and there may be a distinct conflict of interests.

Section 47 of the National Assistance Act 1948

Section 47 of the National Assistance Act 1948, amended 1951, allows for the compulsory removal of an adult from their home under certain circumstances. It states that adults not suffering from mental illness can be placed in an institution compulsorily to 'secure the necessary care and attention' if they:

Are suffering from grave chronic disease or being aged, infirm, or physically incapacitated, are living in insanitary conditions, and

Are unable to devote to themselves and are not receiving from others persons proper care and attention.

The local Public Health Officer applies to a magistrates court for an order committing the person to institutional care, usually either a local hospital or old people's home. If the person is placed in hospital, however, there is nothing in the order that allows for treatment, and treatment can still be refused. Because of its obvious infringements on personal liberty, the use of this Act is declining, and there are great regional variations, with some Local Authorities never using it at all.

Court of protection (public trust office)

This court has responsibility for the financial affairs of people who, through mental impairment, are no longer capable of managing their finances. The Court is an office of the Lord Chancellor's office, and it works by appointing a receiver for the person concerned. This comes under the protection division of the court. There is a management division which will act as the receiver if no other person can be found to do so. The application for the appointment of a receiver can be made by anyone (carer, friend, relative, neighbour or Local Authority), though if it is not the nearest relative that applies, the court will want to know why.

The court usually becomes involved when the person's assets are over £5,000, though it may be interested in people with sums below this, allowing the payments to be made by 'summary order' without a receiver being used. The court supervises the receiver and reviews all transactions to make sure that the finances are being properly managed. Even though the receiver is acting on behalf of the person concerned, the supervision of the court can mean that there are complications, and the court charges for this supervising role. The Lord Chancellor's office also has visitors to help with particular problems. The medical visitors are consultant psychiatrists who assist in difficult decisions as to whether a person can manage financially, make a will (having testamentary capacity). General visitors will call in on clients in various settings, and the visitors from the management division make a yearly visit to those clients for whom the division is acting as receiver.

Power of attorney

In this situation one person, whilst still mentally competent, gives another person the authority to act on their behalf. They usually do this because, although they are still mentally active, they are now too frail to do the actual tasks of going to the bank, paying bills, etc. A power of attorney is a legal document that can be shown to banks and so on (use a copy and leave the original with the legal advisor). It can be cancelled at any time, usually in writing, and it can be general (for day-to-day tasks) or just for a specific transaction (for example, selling a house). Until comparatively recently it became invalid when the person giving the authority became mentally incompetent.

If an elderly person wants the power of attorney to continue after they become mentally frail and finally incompetent, then they must use a different Act, the Enduring Power of Attorney Act 1985. The transfer of powers must occur while the person is still fully mentally alert. There are restrictions to protect the person from exploitation; as the Law Commission put it:

> We have in mind the donor who is no longer fully capable when he grants the Enduring Power of Attorney, even though he still has sufficient capacity to create the power. This is likely to be a very common case in practice where (as will be most usual) the donor is elderly.

Agency

In this case a nominated person (the agent) acts on a frail person's behalf within specific instructions. This is especially seen in the social security system, where a pensioner will nominate someone to collect their benefits from the post office. The agent can only collect the money and then hand it to the person concerned. Many people use this form of help to enable friends, neighbours or home helps to collect pensions.

There is a set procedure for this latter form of transaction. The pensioner deletes 'I acknowledge receipt of the above sum' which is printed on the pension book. They then sign it as usual, and write and sign on the back 'I am unable to go to the post office and I authorise (name)'. This must be signed by the agent and witnessed by someone other than the agent. The agent also has to sign the following: 'I am today the authorised agent. I certify that the payee is alive today. I acknowledge receipt of the amount shown overleaf which I will pay to the payee forthwith'.

Disabled Persons Act 1986

This Act was passed by Parliament in 1986, but its 18 sections are being brought into force gradually. The Act gives disabled people four rights:

- The right to representation – in cases of mental or severe physical incapacity the Local Authority can appoint a representative on behalf of the disabled person or ask a voluntary organisation to appoint someone.
- The right to assessment – this includes any disabled person who asks for services from the Local Authority under Section 2 of the Chronically Sick and Disabled Persons Act 1970.
- The right to information – if a disabled person receives a service from social services then they must also be informed of the other services available and any other relevant services provided by other Local Authorities.
- The right to consultation – the Chronically Sick and Disabled Persons Act 1970 states that certain councils and committees should have a disabled person or someone with special knowledge on that committee. The 1986 Act states that the person can only be appointed after consultation with organisations for disabled people.

The living will

Many people fear becoming old and 'senile' because once they are mentally frail they will no longer be able to tell people what their wishes are, especially in relation to medical treatment. Currently, the position is that doctors dealing with the mentally frail are governed by what is known as 'good medical practice': because the person concerned cannot give consent, measures are taken 'in their best interests'. Most teams of professionals in the United Kingdom would discuss any dilemma with the person's family, although the latter have no legal force to sway the doctors one way or the other (Enduring Powers of Attorney specifically exclude medical matters). 'Good medical practice' may mean that a person undergoes an operation or is given some form of treatment that his family and friends know would have been refused had the person been competent.

In the United States there has been legislation in many states to try to insist on the autonomy of the person under consideration being paramount. To do this, the person must make a statement saying how far they would like the doctors to go in the event of them becoming incapable of giving informed consent. Obviously, such a statement must be made before any brain damage has occurred. This statement is called a living will and describes a form of anticipated consent. The following is an example of a living will:

> It is my express wish that if I develop an acute or chronic cerebral illness which results in a substantial loss of dignity, and the opinions of two independent physicians indicate that my condition is unlikely to be reversible, any separate illness which may threaten my life should not be given active treatment.

The above example is only one type of document that could be drawn up; some people would perhaps want to refuse life support machines or mutilating operation but would want antibiotics or some forms of 'invasive' medical treatment. The United Kingdom is certainly different in its treatment of the very mentally frail, and few doctors here would deem it appropriate to put someone with advanced dementia onto a life support machine or subject them to major operations without the likelihood of significant benefit to the individual. Good medical practice, however, still leaves important decisions in the hands of comparative strangers whose moral and ethical values may differ markedly from those of the person they are treating.

That is not to say that good practice does not currently allow for the extremely mentally frail with other severe illness to die pain-free and with dignity. The British Medical Association (BMA) was initially reluctant to acknowledge the need for living wills, and in the 1980s its Ethics Committee reported that they were quasi-legal documents that could arouse fear in some people. The debate has continued, however, and new impetus has been given to the topic by the large numbers of people affected by AIDS. The Terrence Higgins Trust, a leading AIDS charity, has produced its own living will and distributes copies free of charge. Because AIDS and HIV-related diseases affect a predominantly younger population than dementia, they have focused attention away from age and onto the point at issue, personal autonomy.

The current situation is that living wills are generally considered valid and binding on the medical profession but are not legal documents in the United Kingdom. Doctors are encouraged to respect their contents, and if they have religious or other objections they should transfer the case to a colleague.

The need for discussion of this very important topic is evident. We feel very strongly that many people would contemplate writing a living will to the effect that they would not want their life prolonged in a situation where they will become dependent, simply because currently many institutions caring for the elderly mentally frail are so underfunded and under-staffed that the reality of life in these places fills many people with dread.

Should the living will be legally recognised, funding for services for the elderly must not be cut merely because of a cynically anticipated lack of demand later. The living will debate is only valid if more resources are placed in this sector so that the reality for the elderly mentally infirm in care is an attractive environment, a single room with bath and toilet, and sufficient care staff properly trained to ensure life with dignity. A living will for further possible illness would then truly enhance a person's autonomy.

Do Not Resuscitate (DNR) orders

At home we die, in hospital we have a cardiac arrest: that is, the heart stops. This sudden stopping of the heart can, on occasion, be reversed by the use of cardiac massage (pumping the heart externally) and by applying an electric shock to the chest to try to stabilise the electrical rhythm of the heart again. The most common time for the heart to stop suddenly is after a heart attack, so coronary care units (CCUs) have a higher than average chance of re-starting their patients hearts (the patients in CCU also tend to be younger). The chances of the cardiac arrest team re-starting the heart on a general ward are small. This is because the heart often stops before anyone notices (for example, the person collapses in the toilet and is not found immediately) or the patients tend to be older with many diseases and poorer overall health, making the chances of success less.

On entering hospital the medical team should discuss with each person what their wishes are if their heart should stop unexpectedly. Some people want the cardiac arrest team to try to resuscitate them, others do not. For some people resuscitation is not appropriate, i.e. they are in the last stages of a terminal illness. If the patient cannot have the discussion about whether or not they want them to try and resuscitate them it is good clinical practice to discuss the situation with the nearest relatives or carers.

There is controversy, however, because many doctors find it difficult to raise this issue. This is not surprising. When faced with an ill person, it does not feel comfortable to discuss the possibility of dying. This has led to many doctors making the decision without discussion with the patient; that is, acting in their 'best interests'. For many people this is far too paternalistic, and high-profile cases have hit the press where someone has found on their case notes 'do not resuscitate' or 'DNR' (or other euphemisms such as 'not for 222'). The situation can be especially difficult when considering the patient with dementia. Early disease does not necessarily mean that the person would not want to continue living if at all possible, whereas in late disease it would not be appropriate to consider a cardiac arrest situation leading to a stay in intensive care with no improvement at the end of it.

The principle is, however, that people should be asked and if necessary carers should be involved in coming to a decision. The situation is made harder by the fact that doctors are given very little help in this difficult area. A lot depends on how they explain resuscitation to the patient carers. Too much detail (how the chest is pushed up and down, a tube put into the airway and an electric shock given across the heart) will leave most people declining. A gentle but vague explanation means that people will not really understand what they are consenting to. If the issue is important to an individual or carer, they should raise it with the medical team at the earliest opportunity. If a senior doctor really feels it is inappropriate to attempt the resuscitation process, they cannot be made to do so, but they need to indicate their reasons in the medical notes.

Abuse of elderly people

In the late 1970s articles concerning the physical abuse of elderly people created a flurry of debate and then interest waned. Even though reports have appeared at regular intervals documenting isolated cases and occasionally large-scale institutional abuse, it is the physical and sexual abuse of children that has caught the public imagination and has retained a firm hold on it. The recognition of abuse of older people is probably at the same stage as that of child abuse in the 1970s – the explosion is yet to come.

What is old age abuse? The definitions are varied and range from the broad notion of misuse of power to the more hardened physical or sexual assault. In between are the concepts of emotional, psychological and verbal abuse. What we do know is that there is less research in this field than in that of child abuse. Many consider old age abuse a moral problem, a concern of society, a reflection of its attitudes and concepts of what is acceptable. We know it exists, but there is much debate as to the size of the problem. Some social workers are beginning to take the problem very seriously, and their preliminary studies indicate that up to five per cent of their cases involve some aspect of abuse of an old person. The main areas of abuse can be defined as:

- assault, including forced feeding
- deprivation of nutrition
- misuse of drugs – depravation and overdosing
- emotional/verbal, including intimidation
- sexual
- deprivation of help and aids when disabled
- involuntary isolation
- financial

The abuse of older people is a very complex issue. In one research study a large group of carers agreed to be interviewed. Two-thirds of the group admitted to losing their temper with an elderly relative they cared for, and one-fifth said they occasionally resorted to shaking or hitting the person. One-fifth also reported that the sufferers tried to or did hit them, especially those that were confused, and it was this confused group that were most likely to be hit themselves. The most comprehensive (and only large-scale) survey of elder abuse in the United Kingdom was carried out in 1992. In a random sample of older people it found that five per cent had been verbally abused, two per cent physically abused and two per cent financially abused. The same survey looked at adults in a caring role and found that 10 per cent admitted verbally abusing and one per cent said that they had physically abused an older person.

Research around the world indicates that all older people are at risk of being abused, not only the most frail, most challenging elderly. Much abuse in old age is husband to wife, though it is impossible to say whether these relationships have always involved domestic violence or whether the violence is a new occurrence. Other studies have shown that as many men as women are abused and that, contrary to other violence phenomena, women also perpetrate elder abuse. It was initially assumed, especially in the UK, that most abuse was caused by carer stress. A carer looking after a very challenging older person snaps and hits or hurts the older person in some way. No one condones the behaviour but the basis of the behaviour is understood. Studies in both the US and the UK indicate, however, that carer stress is not a leading cause of abuse. That is not to say that carers are not stressed but that this stress takes its toll in other ways and does not manifest in abuse. It appears that a lot of abuse is due to personality issues in those in a caring role, for example alcohol or drug abuse. In some cases personality disorder or mental health problems predispose to perpetration of abuse, but work in this area is not precise enough to indicate which problems pose most risk.

We do know that carers feel isolated and lonely in their role and that predeterminants to abuse include poor previous relationship, dependency on the older person for money or housing and a real reluctance to be in the caring role in the first place.

People with dementia may be unable to disclose the abuse because of their mental impairment. Memory loss also makes the person with dementia an unreliable witness if the case goes to court. Older people may have a fear of being 'put away' and may live with the abuse, feeling that it is better than the alternative of residential or nursing care. Physical symptoms and signs may indicate to others that something is wrong. An elderly person cowering and obviously frightened of being touched is suspicious. There are no absolute signs, often it is a pattern of features over a period of time that leads to abuse being suspected. Elderly people can bruise easily, with some having the transparent skin syndrome (bruises with minor trauma, due to thinner skin that has been altered by excess sun exposure). Falls can cause older people to have marks on arms and legs. Bruises of different ages and signs of general neglect are worrying, as are thumbprint bruising and bruising in odd places such as the front of the chest (usually protected) and around the jaw and eye or hairline. Delays in seeking help, stories about the injury that do not add up or are different between carer and older person are other pointers. Deterioration in diseases that are usually well controlled on medication can be another indicator that all is not well, as can the older person arriving at hospital, especially if confused, without their carers.

Obviously, abuse is not confined to a domestic setting. It occurs in residential and nursing homes as well as hospitals, day centres and other places. Enough scandals have occurred within these settings to give an outline of what goes wrong. Abusers are able to continue abusing because of a number of issues: colleagues who keep quiet or leave; no effective management scrutinising complaints or problems; no staff education or training process; low wages and poor conditions of service making recruitment of quality staff difficult; and no one listening to residents. Other clues include poor quality markers such as a dirty environment, a rigid regime to suit the workers' needs rather than the clients' and an 'institutional' feel.

Solutions

Elder abuse is a growing area of concern. In 2000 the government produced a report called 'No Secrets'. In it they identified local social service departments as the lead agency in tackling elder abuse. Social services are expected to have liaised with various stakeholders (social workers, police, GPs, hospital doctors, voluntary organisations, etc.) and have developed pathways that clients, carers or workers can access where abuse is suspected. The pathways will include detailed guidelines for approaching and managing a case of suspected abuse, obtaining the story, assessing the risk, immediate management, role of case conferences, etc. If problems or concerns arise regarding institutions, they should be brought to the attention of the relevant manager. If this fails to rectify the situation, a written complaint should be sent to the customer relations department for hospital trusts, the inspection and registration unit of the local health authority for nursing homes, and the registration unit at the local authority for residential homes. Complaints are now taken much more seriously than was formerly the case, and form part of the new health culture of trying to identify risks and respond to them.

The national charity Action on Elder Abuse is an excellent source of educational materials and expertise on this topic, and has a national helpline (see Appendix 2, page 180). This can be used by elderly people as well as carers, relatives and witnesses to abuse of all kinds (for example nurses, care assistants, etc.). The service is free and confidential. Much remains to be done to raise awareness of this issue and to bring help to older people in difficult and upsetting situations. We all have a right to a life free from violence. Older people have a right to be treated with kindness, respect and care in any institutional setting. Carers of all forms need training, guidance and access, where necessary, to further help, especially if the caring role (be it in a domestic situation or in an institution) proves too challenging. Malicious care requires the full force of the law to eradicate it and protect our very vulnerable people.

Driving

Once a diagnosis has been made and a person is deemed to be geographically disorientated in time and place, it is the GP's responsibility to inform the Driver Vehicle License Agency (DVLA). For detailed information see the DVLA website at www.dvla.gov.uk or their advice booklet.

Council Tax

A diagnosis of dementia may exclude the person from payment of Council Tax. A form is available from the Local Authority Council Tax office.

European Union – Human Rights Act

This new legislation looks set to challenge many current practices. It takes a wide perspective on human rights so that many current procedures, actions and laws may be deemed unlawful and banned in the future.

9

Areas of Conflict

In this chapter the potential areas of conflict between sufferer, carer and the medical professionals will be discussed. Two main areas are specifically focused upon:

- obtaining medical help
- discharge from hospital

Obtaining help

For most of us our main medical carer is the General Practitioner. If a medical problem is serious then the GP should see the person at home, especially if the patient is old and somewhat frail. Obtaining this visit should not be difficult. If the person concerned or the carer feels that they cannot get to the surgery, then a GP should visit. In all other instances, unless the GP routinely sees their elderly patients at home, one should try and get to the surgery. Many people complain that they cannot get past the receptionist for either a home visit or a chance to speak to the doctor. The receptionist has a job to do and most manage to find out the problem, fit in appointments, do a host of other things and remain friendly. If, however, you feel you must speak with the doctor then insist on doing so. Most receptionists only protect the doctor so far, and are then under orders to pass the problem on.

Any difficulties with medication should be reported at once so that medicines can be stopped if the GP thinks it advisable. Anyone on repeat prescriptions should see their doctor regularly and have the need for the medicine reassessed. If a hospital appointment changes the medication, be sure to let the GP know, as it sometimes takes many weeks for hospital letters to arrive.

Many elderly people and their carers worry about health issues, but they often keep their worries to themselves. The GP should be told of any concerns so that the person can be listened to, examined and then either reassured or the problem dealt with. No symptom should been taken simply for a sign of old age, especially if the problem involves confusional episodes, falls, incontinence or decreased mobility. The GP can perform many of the screening tests necessary to rule out treatable causes, but may then want to refer the person to a specialist. There is now an ideal opportunity to discuss some of these issues regularly. GPs are now obliged to offer a screening/assessment visit to all elderly people over the age of 75. The GP may visit or invite you to the surgery, or they may delegate the screening to a practice nurse. The areas that have to be asked about are sight, hearing, feet, diet, weight and blood pressure, but an elderly person can add any issue that is worrying them. This can prove to be an excellent time to get one's questions answered.

Many carers feel that their relative was not referred to a specialist soon enough. This dilemma is often a difficult one, for in some cases the specialist cannot offer any more help then is already given. However, in most difficult cases a second opinion is no bad thing and it can at least reassure sufferer and carers that no stone is being left unturned in the effort to help. Most GPs will not refuse a referral to another doctor unless they really feel that it is not justified.

Hopefully, real areas of conflict between patient/carer and doctor will be few, but as a last resort one is entitled to leave one GP's books and join another practice. Help is available from the health authority, Primary Care Trust or Citizens' Advice Bureaux. GPs are not only the gatekeepers to further medical tests and advice; they also can hold sway over the local district nurses and health visitors. Changes in these services often have to go through the GP, but it is worth contacting the services directly if there are any problems.

Some carers report a reluctance on the part of GPs to deal with the acute conditions that can occur in someone with dementia. These acute-on-chronic crises can be very frightening. GPs may see the problem in the light of the underlying dementia, i.e. the fact that the person has one untreatable condition leads to the assumption that all other occurring problems are untreatable. Nothing could be more wrong – acute illnesses resolve in the confused elderly as in other people. What is wrong is to allow an already confused person to become even more disorientated and upset through the clinician's ignorance. In difficult cases it is often possible to ask the GP to arrange for a home visit by an elderly care specialist or psychiatrist of old age. This gives an opportunity for a thorough airing of views and anxieties, and allows the specialist to see the sufferer in their own home, to meet the carer and listen to them, and – hopefully – also to meet the GP at the patient's home and discuss the case.

Respite breaks and holiday breaks are initially arranged through the GP, who then contacts the relevant organisation. Obviously, as much notice as possible should be given. Admission to hospital for whatever reason is usually based on the decision of the GP. Some elderly people are extremely reluctant to consider hospitalisation and need great reassurance; the GP will know of any other schemes that may be available to keep an elderly person at home and yet give them the care that they need. Some areas have 'hospital at home' schemes, with intensive nursing hours provided; on other occasions the local day hospital may be appropriate. New intermediate care schemes are developing (see Chapter 5). Problems do arise when either the person themselves or a carer feels that hospitalisation is necessary but the GP disagrees. This can usually be talked through and a solution agreeable to both parties arrived at, but should there be any medical change in the person's condition then the GP should be called back.

Good GPs are worth their weight in gold; bad ones can mean misery to a frail old person and their carers. Their gatekeeping role is a very powerful one indeed.

Discharge from hospital

This particular area can be fraught with problems and has come to the government's attention. There are now very strict guidelines for hospitals concerning the discharge process and these guidelines must be followed. The ideal should be as follows.

The medical problem is over, the person treated and looking forward to returning home. Any carers involved are happy with the situation and have met with the hospital staff concerning the discharge. Any mobility problems have been identified and a home visit has been carried out by the hospital therapy staff. Prior to discharge the multi-disciplinary team meet and all contribute their views. A care plan is agreed with the patient and family and is written up by the social worker. If this requires a lot of new services, the community care manager either automatically agrees it or calls a case conference. A discharge date is set and each member carries out any special tasks (for example, the ward staff order the ambulance, social worker will arrange the care services, the junior doctor will write a discharge note and organise any medication to go with the patient). Patient and carer are kept informed of all actions as is the GP, and the discharge goes ahead uneventfully. The key is communication.

Unfortunately, many discharges do not resemble the above at all. Many excuses are given, but inevitably the failure is in communication. There are no easy answers, but professionals should not get away with bad practice. If the discharge procedure goes seriously wrong, then the people concerned should know about it. Vigorous complaints are one way to change and hopefully improve the service. No one likes to complain, but without such guided criticism mistakes will continue to occur. Complaining itself is no easy process, but again this has been recognised by the government, and each hospital now has a complaints procedure which should go into action immediately, offering an acknowledgement within four days. To ensure that the problem gets looked into, the complaint must be in writing and preferably addressed to the service manager and/or the hospital's complaints officer (customer services). In very serious cases a copy of the letter should also go to the hospital's Chief Executive. This is not to say that many difficulties cannot be resolved by speaking to the various people concerned, but where a change of practice is needed, a letter is necessary. You should get a reply fully examining your complaint and signed by the Chief Executive within four weeks. If you are not satisfied, you can continue the complaint procedure with the possibility of an Independant Review. If you remain unhappy after that, you may then contact the Health Service Commissioner (ombudsman – see Appendix 2).

A special difficulty occurs when a carer feels that a person cannot return home. This happens extremely frequently, particularly since the recent pressures on NHS and community resources. Often an admission to hospital because of an acute illness becomes a necessary opportunity for total evaluation of the difficulties at home as experienced by the patient and carer. There is always a long history of increasing failure to cope at home, with either no help sought or that help having failed in some way. The situation is at its most desperate where the elderly mentally confused are concerned and the resources are indeed limited. Bear in mind that carers have to be pretty desperate to say no to the massed authority of the hospital hierarchy.

If a carer feels concerned about the impending discharge of a relative, then they must speak out as soon as possible. In many cases discussion with the various team members involved will allow for a compromise, and more help will be provided if possible. If this does not allay fears sufficiently, the carer and other people involved should meet up with the consultant concerned; it may be appropriate to invite others to this meeting, such as the social worker dealing with the case. In cases of real conflict then a case conference should be held, involving the multidisciplinary team as well as the carers, community agencies involved and the person concerned. Carers should ask for such a meeting if they are really unhappy about an impending discharge; it allows everyone to say their piece and the carer in particular to point out the realities of the situation to the other conference members. The point of the conference is to arrive at a solution acceptable to everyone.

Where the patient is able to communicate well, their wishes are paramount, and if they want to return home then as much as possible must be done to ensure that this happens. Often this involves the taking of considerable risks, and carers are sometimes counselled to accept this. Where the patient is mentally frail, however, and not able to vocalise their wishes clearly, the task is harder. The choice is usually between the patient going home against the carer's wishes, and entering some form of institution. These decisions are never easy and there is pressure on both sides. The consultant has a commitment to other people who need the beds and services of the hospital and must take this into account as well as the multidisciplinary team's appraisal of whether or not a return home is feasible. The carers, on the other hand, have often been through it all before. Their concern for a relative may be so great, however, as to cloud their judgement and not allow them to see alternatives. There are no easy answers. The two sides must trust each other, and in most cases a solution is found reasonably amicably. Nevertheless, the equation at the moment is weighted far too heavily in favour of the hospital, and there is a general need for the wishes of the patient and carer to be more forcibly stated and, more importantly, acted upon.

10
Research and the Future

Research into any medical condition requires the participation of patients. Without their help medical research would flounder and we as a society would be critically disadvantaged. If this book is dedicated to anybody it is to the thousands of people who have given of their time and bodies without complaint for the greater good. Memory disorder teams will have a greater and more influential role as therapeutic strategies become available in the UK following on from the National Institute for Clinical Excellence's positive ruling. Additionally, the memory clinic team will be a resource for research and an appropriate base for understanding the role of newer therapies of both a physical and psychological nature.

The use of human subjects in research into dementia is more important than in other areas of research because no animal model exists for Alzheimer's disease, although the so-called 'transgenic' mouse is a useful comparison test animal. It is using this animal that antibodies to amyloid (the protein in brain plaques) have been developed in Edinburgh recently with some success, although human experimentation is still some way off. How best to undertake experimentation into Alzheimer's disease remains problematic.

What next?

Opportunities for research exist in many different areas, not just drug therapies. What is becoming clearer is that cognitive impairment is a problem that affects not only individuals but also families and society at large. Families are increasingly asking about genetic testing (covered in Chapter 4), but this also begs the question of counselling strategies, which are largely missing from NHS provision. Researchers are also attempting to detect very early cognitive decline in the hope that earlier treatment will delay symptomatic disease even longer than is possible at present. The drug companies are particularly interested in care-giver stress and quality of life while patients are being treated, and especially in carer depression. The major question remains, however, what causes Alzheimer's disease in the first place?

Reports of a successful vaccine against AD caused excitement in the scientific community in early 2001. The vaccine induces a specific response against beta-amyloid (the protein that makes up senile plaques) and has been shown to prevent plaque formation in mice. In animal models this vaccine has also been shown to improve cognitive function. The mice used were engineered so that their brains mimicked human ones. The work continues and is especially advanced in North America, although trials in humans are still some way off.

The causes of cognitive impairment

The average GP in the United Kingdom, with a list of 2,000 patients, can expect to have between 20 and 30 patients with dementia. Many will not even come to the attention of the GP, the least affected being the least prominent. However, since the acetylcholinesterase inhibitor drugs have had media coverage, more and more people are presenting earlier, and hitherto undervalued services are becoming inundated with referrals for assessment.

Highly technical explanations are out of place in this text, but it is important to note the areas of opportunity where memory disorder teams may focus in the future to develop strategies for helping clients with memory difficulties:

- familial relationships in dementia
- screening for early memory loss
- legal and ethical issues in the early diagnosis of dementia
- the uses of brain imaging and electrical tracings of brain activity in diagnosis
- biological markers for dementias (blood and spinal fluid)
- new psychological tests for assessment
- new drug treatments
- antibody trials to destroy diseased tissue
- counselling and how to go about this most effectively
- behavioural techniques to modify distressing behaviour
- how to alleviate care-giver burden

Websites can be helpful, since they are continuously updated and provide links to other areas of interest (for useful websites see Appendix 2, page 180). However, searching for impartial information can be tricky. Key in 'Alzheimer's' and around 286,000 pages (and rising) will be listed! And technical names vary: 'galantamine', for example, can also be spelt 'galanthamine'. Searching each spelling brings up different sets of drugs and pages posted by carers or patients. Get what information you can and discuss it with your doctor to reach a balanced conclusion.

Social research

Recently, the strong biological medical focus has been balanced more by research into social phenomena. Making the sufferer more 'accessible' to carers in terms of social interaction has become a goal of pharmacological treatment as well as the focus of some drug company advertising. This is vitally important, since for too long carers have been taken for granted and their needs ignored. More work is also being done to educate professionals who come into contact with elderly people, and especially the elderly mentally confused. Research indicates that, from medical students to politicians, there is a lack of knowledge and interest in the problems of elderly people. The culture we live in is slowly changing as the 'grey vote' is seen as a powerful force for social and medical change in health policy.

The 'big three' possible causes (aetiology)

The remainder of this chapter is information that has been included for those readers who would like to know more about the medical research issues. Clearly, it cannot do justice to the fantastic work that is being undertaken all over the world in highly specialised laboratories. It is hoped, however, that it will give some indication of the possibilities that are being researched with a view to one day developing a cure for a complex and aetiologically elusive disease.

The momentum to effect change in outcome for dementia sufferers is increasing rapidly. Below are listed some of the theories which still play a part in our understanding of the various potential contenders for the root cause of Alzheimer's disease. It is now certain that it is a combination of factors which influence whether a person develops the disease and which sub-type.

- genetic theory
- the aluminium hypothesis
- viral/prion causes

Genetic theory

There have always been some cases of Alzheimer's disease that appears to run in families. The most well researched have been those where the pattern is for younger people to develop the disease. We know, however, that this type of dementia is rare, constituting only around 0.1 per cent of the total number of cases overall. Yet such pre-senile groupings are important in understanding the possible genetic basis for AD, when it runs so prominently in families.

Set against these rare incidences of family occurrences, we know that AD becomes increasingly likely as we age, with over 20 per cent of the over-80s being affected. The question that has perplexed researchers is whether there is a latent genetic fault that leads to the development of the disease, or whether these cases appear 'out of nowhere' as it were. Since, going on current statistical information, most of us will get to the age of 80, then 20 per cent of us will develop the disease based on purely epidemiological grounds.

Clinicians have noticed that people with Down's syndrome develop a condition identical to AD before they die – comparatively young. It had been recognised for a long time that people with Down's syndrome age very quickly, but it was not until the observation was made that they also develop AD that their importance to understanding the genetic model for Alzheimer's was realised. The brains of people with Down's are identical to those of people with late onset AD. We still do not know the causes of AD fully, but we do know those of Down's syndrome: in the majority of cases it is due to an extra chromosome.

Each of us has 23 pairs of chromosomes (the genetic material inherited from each parent), making 46 in total per cell. The only cells in the body with fewer are those of the sperm and the egg, which have 23 each. When Down's syndrome occurs something goes wrong at fertilisation – usually it is duplication of part of chromosome 21, or more rarely a duplication of part of chromosome 14 or 19. It was therefore deduced that a gene on part of chromosomes 21, 19 or 14 led to the genetic origin of Alzheimer's disease. Ultimately the search has resulted in finding a protein created from a gene called apolipoprotein E. This seems to be involved in producing dysfunctional brain metabolism leading to the formation of plaques.

Most researchers do not think that having this gene alone creates a situation where AD will ultimately emerge, merely that it is a highly influential contributing factor in brain pathology. Since carrying the gene does not automatically mean someone will develop AD, the genetic testing of potential sufferers is, to say the least, problematic. Greater attention is now being focused on environmental triggers.

The aluminium hypothesis

Aluminium is found to be at the centre of the 'senile plaques' throughout the brains of AD sufferers, mainly located in the fronto-temporal regions. Attention has been focused on areas of the country where water containing high levels of aluminium, presumably from industrial waste, is to be found. Aluminium is also one of the commonest metals in the earth's crust and a substance used for the production of most household pots and pans. The human body does not require much aluminium in order to perform its various metabolic activities; what is not wanted is excreted in the urine. Problems similar to dementia have been found in renal dialysis patients, who developed extremely high levels of aluminium because dialysis machines were not removing this element routinely. The patients became confused. With newer technology it is possible to remove aluminium more effectively, and dialysis is much safer as a consequence. Since the body excretes all the aluminium it does not need under normal circumstances, the role of high dose aluminium in Alzheimer's remains in doubt; however, as a single cause of AD it is highly unlikely.

Viral/prion causes

We are more certain about the effect of viruses or smaller particulate organisms (prions) which are in the environment and ready to invade our bodies intermittently. Viruses are tiny packages of protein with either DNA or RNA at their core. This allows them to inhabit our bodies, highjack our reproductive cell mechanisms and reproduce themselves with either harmful or benign effects on our constitution. We have all been exposed to viruses, such as the common cold and influenza, that reach us through the air we breathe or, more rarely, as in AIDS or hepatitis, through the blood. There are many varieties of virus, all with different mechanisms for survival and choice of host. Insects, mammal and marine and aquatic life are not immune to their destructive force, and they come in myriad shapes and sizes.

We are unsure of the cause of many disease processes. Some scientists believe that viruses are often to blame, although they have not yet been isolated from damaged tissue. Rheumatoid arthritis and multiple sclerosis are conditions that some suspect have a viral origin. That illnesses including even schizophrenia have a climatic and regional predisposition makes this hypothesis – in the absence of hard evidence – pretty convincing.

Theories that involve animal reservoirs for viruses are commonplace, but absolute evidence has not yet been located. What is really fascinating about viruses is that their effects can be delayed for many years after infection. Herpes viruses and measles can lie low before reeking havoc on the patient. It is the 'slow viruses' that are now coming in for scrutiny.

The new variant CJD (nvCJD) or BSE story

Viruses and prions can cause dementia. The new variant Creutzfelt-Jacob prion (nvCJD) is on the increase and thought to be related to ingesting beef infected with a similar organism causing bovine spongiform encephalopathy (BSE). Although CJD somewhat resembles Alzheimer's, however the infectious agents responsible for the former do not cause the latter. A recent review published in the *British Medical Journal* (April 2001) concluded that new variant CJD causes a brain disease known as a spongiform encephalopathy. This disease is distinct from AD.

Advances in understanding amyloid

Many studies have given support to the idea that 'fibrils' (39-43 amino acid chains) when grouped together as amyloid plaques drive cell destruction in the brain. These plaques have become the hallmark of AD. Other studies have linked inherited, early onset AD to mutations in a forerunner of amyloid (amyloid precursor protein) and other proteins (presenilins 1 and 2) which increase production of the highly 'sticky' Amyloid beta (A beta). The real problem with this theory has been the fact that amyloid plaques often form at some distance from the areas where neuronal cell death is most prominent. It is now thought the smaller soluble toxins which are the component parts of A beta are the missing link. If so, they could provide the crucial target for an AD vaccine.

Psychiatric genetics – new opportunities

If we can understand the basic mechanisms or causes for disease production then two things will naturally follow on. Firstly, there will be improved classification of diseases and secondly, more targeted treatments. Pharmacogenetics is a comparatively new discipline which aims to predict the response and side effects of various treatments based on an individual's genetic make-up (genotype). Several genes have been identified that make an individual more likely to develop AD, and therefore stategies are being devised to help prevent these people from getting the disease.

Gene therapy for neurodegenerative diseases

Scientists involved in this area of research are at the cutting edge of modern medicine. It is still in its infancy and is highly speculative, yet it has produced some startling individual results in some 'incurable' diseases. Broadly speaking, four therapeutic strategies have become available as a direct result of advances in genetics and cell biology:

- **Gene therapy (proper):** delivers healthy genes to a target organ such as the brain. This category includes the specialised field of stem cell transplantation (stem cells are cells derived from embryonic tissue that can potentially develop into any cell in the human body, no matter how specialised it has become, for example nervous tissue).
- **Gene suppression:** aims to reduce the expression of mutated genes, thus preventing the production of harmful products that cells inadvertently engineer.
- **Positional cloning strategies:** identify mutant genes and make use of them for the production of new drugs.
- **Transplantation of (primary) embryonic neural tissue:** used in clinical trials with varying degrees of success, either to improve cognitive function (in Huntington's disease) or motor function (Parkinson's disease).

To date, the first of the above strategies, gene therapy, has only been tested in animal 'models'. The complexities of the experiments have no place in this book, but you will certainly hear a lot more about these exciting developments in relation to AD in the next few years, since what they are attempting to achieve is believed to be within their reach.

Reclassifying the dementias

Recently, medical researchers have begun to look at the microscopic structure of the brain in three conditions that have some obvious similarities but are clinically distinct in presentation and course. These conditions also have some striking similarities when the clusters of symptoms that make up each distinct disease are compared. This has suggested to some doctors that there may be a single basic problem.

It seems that two proteins may be at the root of the problem in three diseases, which can have cognitive impairment as a symptom: Parkinson's disease, multiple system atrophy (Shy-Drager syndrome) and Cortical Lewy Body disease. The two substances are called alpha-synuclein and tau, and make up so-called filamentous inclusions (filaments) within nerve cells which seem to be damaging to the function and structure of nervous tissue. It is the mix or predominance of one or the other substance that makes for the emergence of a distinct clinical picture or disease. It is now being argued that a new system of classification of neuro-degenerative disorders, including the dementias, needs to be established based on the types of destructive proteins found in a sufferer's brain.

New treatments on the horizon

At the time of writing, a new drug is entering the last stages of its clinical development (phase three trial). It is known as Memantine, and is likely to be available in 2003. It is considered to be a neuroprotective agent (it stops the brain being damaged) and is thus different from the current treatments available. Information should be sought from the company developing it (see Appendix 2, page 180). The pharmaceutical company will, like others, produce an Internet resource near the time of its launch.

Conclusions

The late-20th century and early-21st century have seen an enormous interest and real investment into Alzheimer's disease and related conditions. The emerging therapies in the social and medical arenas mean that life for many new sufferers should prove a far cry from the humiliating and nihilistic 'waste bin' into which, sadly, many afflicted with AD were consigned in the past. There is real hope and progress. The momentum to discover a cure is suddenly extraordinary and shows no sign of slowing down.

11

Conclusion

Since the first edition of this book in 1989 much has changed and a lot remains the same. The number of older people in our society has continued to grow and the political goodwill to make older people's lives happier and healthier seems to be more prominent than ever before. The National Service Framework for Older People published in 2001, is evidence of the political commitment to improve quality and access to services. Specialist mental health services have been developing as a real force in health and social services, and their aims to be comprehensive, accessible and multidisciplinary are being realised on the ground. Certainly these services are more individual and systematic than at any other time in the history of the NHS. However, the cost of dementia care alone is estimated at £6 billion a year, and a recent Audit Commission survey indicated that the range of services for older people was highly variable from area to area. The problems that face all of us will only be overcome with a close degree of partnership.

Being old should be seen as a success story. The fact that older people are more prone to a greater number of medical and social problems should not detract from this success. Most elderly people lead fit and independent lives. For those who fall ill much can be done, and for most the illness can be cured or substantially alleviated. Chronic conditions by their very nature will always be with older people in one form or another, but to accept that these conditions inevitably lead to dependence is wrong and should be challenged by those who have the power to advocate independence.

Active rehabilitation, including the newer treatments for dementia, can postpone dependence, perhaps indefinitely for some. Health problems in older people must be treated with as much vigour as those in the young, making old age a time of enjoyment and activity. There will always be some for whom early and accurate diagnosis, full treatment and rehabilitation will be insufficient and in whom the underlying disease process will continue. This remains true of Alzheimer's disease and the other dementias, even in the presence of treatment that slows the disease or helps the symptoms, which are so disabling.

Professor Bennett commented in this chapter over 10 years ago: 'It is to be hoped that, with continuing public and professional education, "ageism" in all areas diminishes. It is morally wrong and financially absurd to spend vast sums of money on a large group of people at the end of their disease process, placing them in institutions instead of ensuring prevention and early detection of disease'. This new edition of this book goes some way towards empowering those who do not know how to ask for help, and gives them most of the information they need to get the help to which they are entitled. Elderly people are no less valuable than people of any other age group, but they remain a comparatively inconspicuous population. The 'grey' vote is increasingly politically important, and older people and government are coming to realise this. Part of this new awareness is leading to more preventative work and early recognition of disease in primary care and general practice. GPs are the gatekeepers of the NHS and should be the first port of call, but if you do not get satisfaction the Community Mental Health Teams are an avenue for accessing services. It is important to remember that policies for assessment will vary from area to area. In addition, NHS Direct now provides medical advice 24 hours a day, seven days a week. This is a useful but as yet unaudited service.

It is hoped that the glossy magazines will soon carry articles on age-related issues as well as on how to stay young and glamorous. All of us will age, but information about confusion is not as available as that about cosmetics. It should be. To many it seems that today's 'youth' society is not listening to how difficult it is to cope with dementia or confusion, but people in old age medicine are listening and are more than willing to help – even if getting through the door can at times seem impossible. Knowing what to do in what circumstances and where to go for practical help and advice is vital. Patients and carers need a network of informal and formal help, and should not be left to cope alone, which is a burden impossible to sustain.

Carers continue to care, even though the sacrifices are enormous in both time and tolerance, but they may only continue to do so if they are met halfway by the state and services for healthcare provision. The voluntary sector is no longer the mainstay of support for many elderly people and their carers, but statutory services still have to convince a sceptical public that they are truly geared up and ready to help unconditionally. Ultimately, the role of carer must be rewarded. Financial help must be widened and the burden recognised in the form of assistance such as respite holidays. The health and social services alone cannot match what a loving carer has to offer. Medicine and psychiatry for older people, for too long the Cinderella disciplines, have come of age. It is time for us all to go to the ball – a lifetime's work has given us admission rights. The future can be brighter for those with dementia.

Appendix 1

Incontinence

It is helpful to look at incontinence as being either voluntary or involuntary; that is to say, the person either knows that they need to pass urine or faeces (and then doesn't do it in the right place), or the person is unaware of this need. The following list outlines the main causes of both conditions:

- Voluntary incontinence of urine
  - immobility
  - confusion
  - environment
  - culture
- Voluntary incontinence of faeces
  - immobility
  - environment
  - culture
- Involuntary incontinence of urine
  - urinary tract infection
  - stress (muscle weakness) incontinence
  - constipation
  - atrophic vaginitis in women (dry and sore front passage due to hormone lack)
  - vaginal prolapse in women (womb dropping down)
  - prostate enlargement in men (swollen gland near bladder causing obstruction)

- retention of urine (full bladder leaking slightly due to prostate gland and constipation in men and infection and constipation in women)
- drugs (for example, diuretics)
- unstable bladder
- Involuntary incontinence of faeces
  - constipation
  - haemorrhoids (piles)
  - rectal fissure (painful crack at the opening of the back passage)
  - rectal tumour (cancer of the back passage)
  - neurological causes (loss of sensation and control in this area)
  - drugs (for example, those which cause a loose stool)

Voluntary incontinence of urine

As the bladder fills with urine, a stage is reached when we realise that we could pass urine if we wanted to and if it was appropriate, but at this stage the need to urinate is non-urgent – we can suppress the sensation, for example if sitting in the cinema or on the bus. Some time later, however, another sensation tells us that we have to go *soon*. Gradually the feeling gets more urgent and painful. If stuck in a lift or tied to a chair, all of us would inevitably have to pass urine, i.e. be voluntarily incontinent. We would know that this was happening, but would be unable to do anything about it.

A person with Alzheimer's disease in a strange environment will suffer this latter fate; they know they need to go but often cannot communicate this or else they can't find a toilet. The person is then either incontinent or they pass urine in an unacceptable place (sink, wastebin, etc.). Carers and others often know when the toilet is needed because the sufferer gets a little more agitated, begins to get up and wander and may clutch their private parts. Guiding them to a toilet quickly is often sufficient. The environment is thus extremely important, not only for the mentally confused but also the other main group that are prone to voluntary incontinence, the immobile. A person with a physical handicap (such as the result of a stroke) will find the stairs up to or down to a public toilet as daunting as you or I would find climbing Everest. A poorly designed environment can mean misery to people with disability and a loss of bladder control.

Drugs (especially diuretics) can cause sudden incontinence. The strong-acting ones begin to work within minutes and fill the bladder so quickly that the incontinence starts before the person is really aware of it, especially if they are a little confused and perhaps slightly immobile. Some people sit on the toilet for a good few hours after taking their tablets, until the danger of incontinence has worn off. It is simpler and better to see one's doctor and change the medication.

We should perhaps remember that for millions of people passing urine when and where they like is a fact of life and as culturally accepted as our use of toilets with all mod cons.

Voluntary incontinence of faeces

This is much less common than voluntary incontinence of urine, but the same basic principles as above apply. It is easy enough to ignore the desire to have one's bowels open, and eventually the urge can go away (the motions move back up the large bowel). However, if this is done frequently then the motions will dam up and get passed involuntarily.

Confusion is one of the main causes of voluntary incontinence of faeces, and providing an easily accessible toilet the best way of treating it. Thus the environment and immobility also play an important role. Again, cultural differences spring to mind – in some countries faeces form the basis of manure in the fields and are passed accordingly.

Involuntary incontinence of urine

The most common cause of this, especially in elderly women, is a urinary infection in the urine (see Chapter 2, page 20). Severe or repeated infection may mean that the infection has gone further up the urinary tract (to the bladder and kidneys) or that there is some abnormality (stones or tumour) in the bladder or kidneys themselves.

Many women suffer from stress or urge incontinence. This is often the result of childbirth, where the muscles around the bladder have been stretched and so cannot keep the opening tightly closed. Usually this means that the person wets themselves if they cough, laugh or strain (so losing some control over the muscles trying to keep the bladder opening closed). Some women, however, have muscles so weak that they wet themselves when they stand up. The same weakness can cause a prolapse, in the most severe cases of which the womb drops down and can be seen. Usually a prolapse is not this bad, but an still cause incontinence.

When constipation is a problem the hard motions in the back passage can push against the bladder and make it pass water. If the bulk of the motion is very big, then the pressure can stop the bladder emptying at all and the bladder fills up (retention). This can happen acutely and can be very painful. In this situation the obstruction must be removed quickly. Occasionally this process happens more slowly and the full bladder keeps going by emptying a little at a time, i.e. the person leaks urine almost continuously. This is a big problem in men because the prostate gland sits at the bottom of the bladder and it commonly gets bigger as men get older. A stage is reached where it begins to cause symptoms (the passing of small amounts of water frequently and with difficulty) and then it can block off the exit to the bladder in the same way as extreme constipation can.

A woman's vagina (front passage) and the tube (urethra) leading up to and just into the bladder is covered by a delicate lining that needs female hormones to keep it moist and supple. In some women after the menopause the hormone levels drop so low that the lining becomes dry and painful and more liable to infections. The bladder opening is also affected and the closing mechanism (sphincter) weakens so that the woman may be incontinent of urine. The application of hormone creams or the taking of hormone tablets relieves this condition.

Another common cause of incontinence of urine is known as the unstable bladder. As described before, the bladder fills up with urine, and as it does so we receive messages telling us how full it is. Only when we are ready (within limits) do all the openings relax and the bladder contracts, pushing out urine. All these actions take place because the nerves around the bladder use chemical messengers to tell the muscles to relax and contract. In the unstable bladder these chemicals are faulty and the bladder begins to contract when it has only a smallish amount of urine in it and before it has told the brain that it is ready – indeed, before the person is ready. This condition appears to occur more commonly in those suffering from dementia, but can occur in anyone (women more than men). The classic tale is of a carer taking someone to the toilet, where they remain for quite a while, then on the way out or just back in the living room the person is incontinent. The incontinence appears wilful but is not. This condition can be diagnosed from the history and the absence of other causes, but usually a cystometrogram is done. In this test a small catheter (tube) is passed into the bladder and another into the back passage. The bladder is filled with water. In an unstable bladder contractions can be soon occurring too soon. Some exercises and drugs appear to help a lot, but mainly in the unconfused group, as co-operation with the treatment is necessary.

Drugs, as mentioned before, can put a great strain on the bladder. Diuretics are the main culprits. These can be either strong, for example loop diuretics containing frusemide or bumetanide, or weak – the thiazides.

Involuntary incontinence of faeces

This is always a serious problem, because it is so unpleasant for both sufferer and carer. But in most cases it is treatable, although this is often not realised. By far and away the most common cause is constipation. This is true whether or not the person has been incontinent of solid motion or of more liquid stools. If someone doesn't open their bowels for a long time the motion in the back passage can get very hard and can dam back a long way, so much so that it can reach part of the bowel where the motions are still liquid. This liquid motion then runs down the outside of the hard stool and leaks out as diarrhoea. If the constipation is very bad the hard motion pushes down and keeps the anus open so that both solid and liquid stools keep being passed. At this stage the bowels must be cleared with enemas or manually, and then a regular bowel habit arranged.

There may be a reason why the person has been trying not to open their bowels (apart from confusion and not finding the toilet). For this reason when faecal incontinence occurs, all people must have their back passage examined – a rectal examination is quick and straightforward. There may be an obvious painful condition, such as piles or a fissure. In the latter condition a small crack appears at the opening of the back passage. This gets inflamed and then causes a lot of pain when a motion is passed; it can be helped with creams, but often needs a small operation to cure it.

Sometimes the examination will reveal a growth in the back passage. These are often painless and cause serious trouble only late in their development. In the early stages they may bleed a little or cause constipation and then diarrhoea intermittently. Faecal incontinence is not usually a problem until a growth is at a late stage. All growths in the back passage must be biopsied (a small piece of the tumour taken for laboratory examination) and analysed under the microscope to see if it is cancerous or not.

Drugs can also cause faecal incontinence. Liquid paraffin is still used as a softener and laxative, but the paraffin can leak out of the back passage and cause incontinence. Some laxatives, for example senna preparations, stimulate the bowel and can be quite strong, causing colic and the sudden passage of a stool, and hence incontinence. Diarrhoea is a potent cause of faecal incontinence because the person may get very little warning of the need to pass a motion and be unable to hold on to the liquid. The following drugs are well-recognised causes of loose motions:

- iron preparations
- laxatives
- antibiotics
- white stomach medicine (magnesium hydroxide)

If none of the above conditions are found to be the cause of the faecal incontinence, then the person should be seen by a specialist, as there are some neurological causes that may respond to treatment. Specialised investigations are often performed and treatment plans given. Faecal incontinence must never be accepted and put down to either age or confusion.

Incontinence aids

Following a full assessment, including toileting regimes and perhaps some behaviour therapy, there will be a residual group of men and women who need aids to help them keep dry/clean and dignified. Very few people should be faecally incontinent after a full assessment, but in severe dementia faecal incontincence may be unavoidable. It is possible to constipate the sufferer with tablets, for example codeine phosphate, and then give them regular enemas, usually twice a week (given by the carer or a district nurse). This seems to work well with many elderly people. New rectal plugs are being developed (see opposite). Alternatively, pads can be used to cope with faecal (and urinary) incontinence.

District nurses and continence advisors are the experts in the field of incontinence and should be approached to discuss the various products available. Carers should ask their GP to arrange a meeting and an assessment.

Incontinence aids for men

Penile pouch	If the problem is occasional slight leakage.
Penile sheath	The sheath is like a condom – it stretches over the penis and is then fastened. A tube collects the urine, which passes into a bag, usually taped to the leg.
Indwelling catheter	A tube is passed via the penis into the bladder, and a small balloon on the end is inflated to keep it there. Urine drains down the tube and into the bag.
Absorbent pads	These are fitted inside leak-proof pants with elasticated sides.
Absorbent sheets	Placed under the person when in bed. They can be washed and reused.

Consider bladder-specific medication in some people.

Incontinence aids for women

Indwelling catheter	A tube is passed up the urethra into the bladder, and urine passes down the tube into a bag. The catheter is shorter than a male catheter and has a smaller balloon.
Absorbent pads	As for men
Absorbent sheets	As for men

Faecal incontinence aids

A new product, a rectal sponge, has recently been developed by Coloplash. A soft plug is inserted gently into the rectum, where it allows gas to pass but not liquid stool (as can occur in faecal incontinence). The plug is removed by pulling a short string when it is convenient to allow the person's bowels to be opened.

Appendix 2

Useful Information, Websites and Further Reading

Organisations providing support and advice:

Action on Elder Abuse
Astral House
1268 London Road
London SW16 4ER
Tel: 020 8764 7648
Elder Abuse Response Helpline: 080 8808 8141
Fax: 020 8679 4074
www.elderabuse.org
Email: aea@ace.org.uk

International Network for the Prevention of Elder Abuse
(INPEA)
www.inpea.net
For information on international issues of abuse.

Alzheimer Research Forum
www.alzforum.org
This website's information database consists of a professional and non-professional section with links to websites
on patient care, support groups, commercial products,

news and general information about the disease, as well as associations and disease centres.

Alzheimer's Society
45–6 Lower Marsh
London SE1 7RG
Tel: 0845 300 0336
www.alzheimers.org.uk
Support and advice on all forms of dementia.

Arthritis Care
18 Stephenson Way
London NW1 2HD
Helpline: 0808 800 4050

British Heart Foundation
Tel: 020 7935 0185
www.bhf.org.uk

Cancer BACUP
Tel: 0808 800 1234
www.cancerbacup.org.uk
Information for patients, relatives and friends.

Multiple Sclerosis Society
Tel: 0808 800 8000
www.mssociety.org.uk
Information and many support services.

National Osteoporosis Society
PO Box 10
Radstock,
Bath BA3 3YB
Tel: 01761 471 771 (general enquiries)
Helpline: 01761 472 721
Email: info@nos.org.uk

Parkinson's Disease Society
Tel: 0808 800 0303 (Mon–Fri, 9.30am–5.30pm)
www.parkinsons.org.uk
Information, advice and support for people with Parkinson's, their carers and care professionals.

Pharmaceutical companies who have developed or are developing drug treatments for dementia:

Janssen-Cilag Ltd (Galantamine)
www.janssen-cilag.co.uk

Novartis (Riverstigmine)
www.HealthandAge.com

Pfizer/Eisai (Donepezil)
www.eisai.co.uk

Lundbeck (Memantine)
www.memantine.com

Government organisations and public health information:

Commission for Health Improvement
www.doh.gov.uk/chi

Department of Health
www.doh.gov.uk

Health Service Commissioner (Ombudsman)
www.ombudsman.org.uk

National Health Service
www. nhs.uk

National Institute for Clinical Excellence
www.nice.org.uk

NHS Direct
Tel: 0845 4647
www.nhsdirect.nhs.uk

Further reading

Bennett G.C.J., Kingston P., *The Dimensions of Elder Abuse*, Macmillan, 1997.

Cayton, Harry, Nori, Dr Graham, Warner, Dr James, *Alzheimer's at Your Fingertips*, Class Publishing, 1997.

Forsythe, Dr Elizabeth, *The Mystery of Alzheimer's: A Guide for Carers*, Kyle Cathie, 1996.

Health Education Authority, *Who Cares? Information and Support for the Carers of Confused People*.

Lay, Chris, Woods, Bob, *Caring for the Person with Dementia: A Guide for Families and Other Carers*, Alzheimer's Disease Society, 1994.

Index